Get Through MRCOG
Part 3

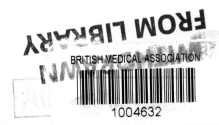

Get Through

Our bestselling *Get Through* series guides medical postgraduates through the many exams they will need to pass throughout their career, whatever their specialty. Each title is written by authors with recent first-hand experience of the exam, overseen and edited by experts in the field to ensure each question or scenario closely matches the latest examining board guidelines. Detailed explanations and background knowledge will provide all that you need to know to get through your postgraduate medical examination.

For more information about this series, please visit: https://www.crcpress.com/Get-Through/book-series/CRCGETTHROUG

Get Through MRCOG
Part 3
Clinical Assessment

Second Edition

T. Justin Clark, MD (Hons), FRCOG
Consultant Gynaecologist and Honorary Professor, Birmingham
Women's & Children's Hospital and University of Birmingham,
Birmingham, UK

Arri Coomarasamy, MD, FRCOG
Professor of Gynaecology, Institute of Metabolism and Systems
Research, University of Birmingham, and Director of Tommy's
National Centre for Miscarriage Research, Birmingham, UK

Justin Chu, PhD, MRCOG, MBChB
Academic Clinical Lecturer and Obstetrics and Gynaecology
Specialist Registrar, University of Birmingham, and Birmingham
Women's & Children's Hospital, Birmingham, UK

**Paul Smith, PhD, MRCOG, MBChB (Hons)
BSci (Hons)**
NIHR Post Doctoral Research Fellow and Obstetrics and Gynaecology
Specialist Registrar, University of Birmingham, and Birmingham
Women's & Children's Hospital, Birmingham, UK

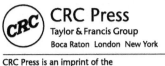

CRC Press
Taylor & Francis Group
Boca Raton London New York

CRC Press is an imprint of the
Taylor & Francis Group, an **informa** business

CRC Press
Taylor & Francis Group
6000 Broken Sound Parkway NW, Suite 300
Boca Raton, FL 33487-2742

Printed on acid-free paper

International Standard Book Number-13: 978-1-138-49847-1 (Hardback)
International Standard Book Number-13: 978-1-138-49846-4 (Paperback)

Visit the Taylor & Francis Web site at
http://www.taylorandfrancis.com

and the CRC Press Web site at
http://www.crcpress.com

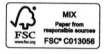

Printed and bound in Great Britain by
TJ International Ltd, Padstow, Cornwall

To Christine, Laura, Alice, Joe and Eleanor
TJC

To Dukaydah, Abdea, Tara and Leela
AC

Dedicated to Anneke and Lily – for their continuing love and support
JJC

I would like to dedicate this book to Rima Smith for her support and laughter
PS

CONTENTS

CONTENTS

PREFACE

Get through MRCOG Part 2 OSCE won a BMJ book award and has been one of the best-selling O&G revision titles over the last decade. We have updated this book to incorporate feedback from over 1000 delegates that have attended our successful MRCOG OSCE course since its inception in 2006 (www.acecourses.co.uk), as to what is needed to pass the MRCOG clinical examination. Furthermore, this successful book has been rewritten to reflect the changes to the OSCE component of the MRCOG that were implemented in 2016, so that this updated book reflects the requirements of the new exam format.

This book mirrors the methods and approaches that we use in the design and delivery of the face-to-face practical course. It benefits from years of feedback regarding the techniques that we teach and the changing RCOG curriculum. Most importantly, this book is not yet another MRCOG Part 3 book with lots of example OSCE stations. Instead, this book focuses on the strategies and techniques that make particular candidates stand out from the rest and perform well for the purposes of the OSCE circuit.

One of the commonest remarks we hear from the candidates attending our course is, *'My Consultants tell me that I am a good clinician, and that I will be fine for the OSCE'*. But what does this statement actually mean? True, for the MRCOG to have clinical credibility, it should discriminate between clinically competent and less proficient candidates. However, with the high number of role-play stations in the new format of the MRCOG Part 3 OSCE, how can a candidate demonstrate that they are a good clinician? If you are told that you are a good clinician, does this mean you do not need to prepare any further for the exam? We would suggest that preparation and having a strategy for each type of OSCE station is a necessity if a candidate is to pass the OSCE. A candidate must have an approach to perform well in every station, such as where they are required to break bad news or to empathise with an angry patient. Similarly, a candidate must not overlook fundamental clinical skills. They should have a reliable and practised structure to take a patient history. They must be able to formulate as well as communicate a management plan. Preparation for all types of OSCE station, likely to be encountered in the MRCOG Part 3, will help performance on the day to be as near perfect as possible.

Other common questions that we are asked can be very basic such as: *'How should we enter the station?'*; *'Should we address the examiner?'*; *'What should I do if everything is going wrong?'* Other questions are more technical, such as *'How do I explain a karyotypical problem?'*; *'How can I show that I teach effectively to medical students?'* The answers to all of these questions are in this book.

We hope that you find every page in this book useful and implement the advice, structures and strategies in it for your preparation for the MRCOG Part 3 OSCE. The contents of this book should empower you to show the skills that you use in everyday clinical practice and will therefore maximise your chances of achieving Membership of the Royal College of Obstetricians and Gynaecologists.

ACKNOWLEDGEMENT

We thank Dr Pallavi Latthe for writing the sample data interpretation station on urodynamics in Chapter 4.

A&E	accident and emergency	**GU**	genitourinary
APH	antepartum haemorrhage	**hCG**	human chorionic gonadotrophin
ARM	assisted rupture of membranes	**HDU**	high dependency unit
ATA	ask, tell and ask	**HPV**	human papilloma virus
BMI	body mass index	**HRQL**	health-related quality of life
BMJ	British medical journal	**HRT**	hormone replacement therapy
BNA	borderline nuclear abnormality	**HVS**	high vaginal swab
BSO	bilateral salpingo-oophorectomy	**ICSI**	intracytoplasmic sperm injection
CBT	cognitive behavioural therapy	**IHD**	ischaemic heart disease
CI	confidence interval	**IMB**	intermenstrual bleeding
COC	combined oral contraceptive	**IMRAD**	introduction, methods, results and discussion
CRL	crown-rump length		
C/S	caesarean section	**IOL**	induction of labour
CT	computerised tomography	**IUCD**	intrauterine contraceptive device
CTG	cardiotograph		
CVA	cerebrovascular accident	**IUGR**	intrauterine growth retardation
CVP	central venous pressure		
DMPA	depo medroxyprogesterone acetate	**IVU**	intravenous urogram
		LH	luteinising hormone
DOA	detrusor overactivity	**LFT**	liver function test
DUB	dysfunctional uterine bleeding	**LMP**	last menstrual period
		LMWH	low molecular weight heparin
ECV	external cephalic version	**LOA**	left occipito-anterior
EFW	estimated foetal weight	**LUS**	lower uterine segment
ERPC	evacuation of retained products of conception	**MDT**	multidisciplinary team
		MRI	magnetic resonance imaging
FBC	full blood count	**MRSA**	methicillin-resistant *Staphylococcus aureus*
FFP	fresh frozen plasma		
FHR	foetal heart rate	**MSU**	midstream urine
FSH	follicle stimulating hormone	**NAD**	no abnormality detected
GA	general anaesthesia	**NNT**	number needed to treat
GIT	gastrointestinal tract	**NTD**	neural tube defect
G&S	group and save	**NVD**	normal vaginal delivery
GTT	glucose tolerance test	**O&G**	obstetrics and gynaecology

OA	occipito-anterior	**RR**	relative risk
OCP	oral contraceptive pill	**SFA**	seminal fluid analysis
OP	occipito-posterior	**SFH**	symphysial fundal height
OSCE	oral structured clinical examination	**SPD**	symphysis pubis dysfunction
OT	occipito-transverse	**STI**	sexually transmitted infection
PCB	post-coital bleeding		
PCO	polycystic ovaries	**TAH**	total abdominal hysterectomy
PID	pelvic inflammatory disease	**TOP**	termination of pregnancy
PMB	post-menopausal bleeding	**TVT**	transvaginal tape
PMH	past medical history	**U&E**	urea and electrolytes
PMS	premenstrual syndrome	**UDCA**	ursodeoxycholic acid
POP	progestogen-only pill	**USS**	ultrasound scan
PPH	postpartum haemorrhage	**VBAC**	vaginal birth after caesarean section
RCT	randomised controlled trial		
RDS	respiratory distress syndrome	**VE**	venous embolism
RPOC	retained products of conception	**VI**	virgo intacta
		VTE	venous thromboembolism

INTRODUCTION

Congratulations on passing your MRCOG Part 1 and Part 2 exams. Success in these two exams is itself a huge achievement as your knowledge of obstetrics and gynaecology and its application in modern-day practice have been tested to a great depth. Your basic science has been rigorously tested in the MRCOG Part 1 exam. Whilst your clinical knowledge has been tested in the SBAs and the clinical application of this knowledge has been tested in the EMQs in the MRCOG Part 2. However, your skills, attitudes, competencies and behaviours in clinical scenarios are yet to be examined. These higher attributes are what the MRCOG Part 3 exam assesses.

It is often suggested that the examiners in the MRCOG Part 3 circuit are trying to answer the following question: Would I want this candidate as my registrar? With the addition of stations implementing lay examiners and role-players having a say on the assessment of each candidate, examiners are also identifying candidates that they would want as their obstetrician or gynaecologist. Therefore, the focus of the OSCE is not to once again test your knowledge but instead to test performance in clinical scenarios and how you can communicate with patients and colleagues. Your holistic, caring and safe approach to medicine is what is being assessed.

Rather than an Objective Structured Clinical Examination (OSCE), the RCOG now call the MRCOG Part 3 exam a Clinical Assessment. The objectiveness remains in the new format of the exam; however, one could argue that the new format is less structured than the old. Instead of having structured marking schemes for clinical examiners to complete, there are five domains that each task can be assessed on. These are:

1. Patient safety
2. Communication with patients and their relatives
3. Communication with colleagues
4. Information gathering
5. Applied clinical knowledge

Three or four of these domains will be assessed in each task and candidates are marked as a pass, a fail or a borderline. Examiners are asked to justify their decision by writing free text. In most tasks, the domains that are being tested will be obvious; however in some tasks, the domains may be more difficult to discern. This is why we believe that developing a strategy for each type of task is required in order to demonstrate proficiency in all of the domains that are being assessed.

The circuit itself comprises 14 task stations with each task representing one of the 14 modules in the MRCOG syllabus (https://www.rcog.org.uk/en/careers-training/mrcog-exams/part-3-mrcog-exam/part-3-mrcog-syllabus/). Each task lasts 12 minutes with an initial 2-minute reading time. Therefore, the total duration of the exam is 168 minutes (almost 3 hours).

There are only two types of tasks: a role-play task (with a patient or colleague) and a structured discussion task. Two tasks out of the 14-task circuit may be linked to each other, and it is expected that candidates build on knowledge acquired from the first task.

This book has been written to help you pass the exam. To provide and teach you the techniques required to perform well in the different types of tasks. The professional and lay examiners are seeking to identify the candidates whom they would want to work with or be looked after. Therefore, if the exam is valid, it should be passed by all able, communicative and caring doctors. If you are one of these doctors, then with the preparation provided in this book, you should be able to obtain your Membership of the Royal College of Obstetricians and Gynaecologists. We wish you the best of luck.

SECTION I
PREPARATION FOR THE MRCOG
PART 3

CHAPTER 1
PREPARATION
FOR THE MRCOG
PART 3

Being a good clinician is not enough to get you through the MRCOG Part 3 exam. We know many young doctors that have surprisingly failed this exam who we feel are excellent clinicians. The correct approach and preparation are required for any exam. But what is the correct approach? And what is the 'right way' to prepare? Some of the aspects of the 'right way' to prepare are detailed in the text that follows.

The 'wrong way' to approach this exam is to prepare how you did for the MRCOG Part 2 exam. Simply put, the MRCOG Part 2 and Part 3 exams are completely different exams with completely different formats and emphases. Therefore, it makes no sense to focus on rebuilding your knowledge again by reading your long MRCOG Part 2 texts. You must remember that this exam assesses your clinical skills, communication, attitudes and behaviours. Knowing the 15 causes of hydrops fetalis is not going to be of benefit. However, a word of caution, you must maintain a steady level of clinical knowledge as this will ensure that you come across as a confident clinician and allow you to communicate true facts to role-players. So, to use the previous example, it may be useful to be aware of three or four causes of hydrops.

PRACTICAL PREPARATION

Know your exam

You must ensure that you are familiar with the format of the Task Circuit. Talk to friends and colleagues that have recently sat the exam. Talk to your senior colleagues who may be MRCOG examiners and read the MRCOG Part 3 syllabus, FAQs and format information provided on the RCOG website (www.rcog.org.uk/en/careers-training/mrcog-exams/part-3-mrcog-exam/part-3-mrcog-syllabus/). We would strongly encourage you to attend an MRCOG Part 3 course; it is certainly beneficial to go through past exam questions with your revision buddy, but going through an actual circuit provides an invaluable preparatory experience. Familiarising yourself in this way with what to expect on the day can also help you maintain focus, provide motivation to 'get over this last hurdle' and afford you the opportunity to share experiences and exchange ideas with peers.

Know your syllabus

The Task Circuit is 14 stations long. Each station assesses you on the 14 modules in the syllabus. Before the exam, you should have a sound understanding of the syllabus.

Develop and stick to a strategy

Sit with your colleagues from around your deanery and design a realistic revision timetable and strategy. We believe that you need at least one revision buddy. Ideally, you would have two for useful practice at mock stations. One person would act as the candidate, one would act as the examiner and the last can act as the role-player. The more practice that you can get through, the better you are likely to perform on the day of the exam. The design of an achievable schedule for practice with your revision buddies is required and should be one of the first things you do, as you will have to coordinate your preparation with your clinical commitments which can be difficult with different shift patterns and on-call duties. Ideally, you should set out short, frequent and focused meetings, and the predominant component should be practising Task Stations.

Study groups or partners

Preparing for this exam on your own can be a lonely experience. If there are no other trainees that are sitting the MRCOG Part 3 at the same time as you, try and ask colleagues to help you do practice stations. Do this early.

We would recommend studying in a group with other candidates of a similar standard to you. The ideal number of candidates working together is three or four. If there are more, then potentially some individuals may not be exposed as the active candidate for any of the practice stations. The benefit of working in a group of three or four is that you can pick up tips from others in the group and learn from their good or bad performances. Working in a group can also maintain a high level of motivation and commits your time to revision.

When meeting in a group, ensure that you set an agenda at the start of the session. Be clear, in which type of stations that you will practise and in how many stations each of you will be the active candidate. Importantly, try and emulate the exam conditions by keeping to time and using a structured marking sheet using a selection of the assessment domains.

Choose your learning materials carefully

Assemble all of your revision materials early and have them ready for when you practise so that you use your time efficiently. In particular, avoid the heavy texts that you have used for the MRCOG Part 2 exam. Instead, we would recommend that you compile your study materials from the following:

1. Patient information leaflets
2. Executive summaries from RCOG guidelines, DFSRH guidelines and relevant NICE guidance
3. A good MRCOG Part 3 exam revision book (like this one!!)
4. Recent BJOG and TOG reviews on topics not covered by guidance
5. The latest MBRRACE-UK report

Arrange meetings with the multidisciplinary team

There will be certain aspects of obstetrics and gynaecology that you are very familiar with. These are topics that you cover during your day-to-day clinical duties such as labour ward management and early pregnancy complications. Inevitably, however, there will be areas with which you are less familiar and that you may have simply had to learn from a textbook or other written sources. To mitigate against this lack of clinical experience, we would recommend that early on in your preparation you try and arrange some meetings with the following people:

- A *paediatrician/neonatologist* – Have a list of topics that you want them to teach you. Ask them to take you through the newborn baby examinations, assessment of neonatal jaundice and neonatal resuscitation, for example.
- A *theatre nurse* – Ask them to take you through commonly used surgical instruments and endoscopic equipment.
- *Specialist midwives* – Some midwives provide specialist services to women. These include women with medical conditions (e.g. diabetes, haemoglobinopathies); vulnerable women often with complex social factors (e.g. substance abuse, teenage pregnancies, obesity, child protection), antenatal/newborn screening services, infant feeding and bereavement/pregnancy loss support. Ask if you can sit in a clinic and observe their work and consultations. Pay particular attention to how they explain things to couples and ask them what phrases they choose to use in particularly difficult situations.
- A *fetal medicine consultant* – Ask them how they describe some of the more common congenital conditions such as congenital diaphragmatic hernia, gastroschisis, Down's syndrome, Patau's syndrome and Edward's syndrome (and their screening).
- A *urogynaecologist* – Many candidates may not be familiar with diagnostic investigations such as urodynamics. Ask them to go through the process of diagnostics and management options for urinary incontinence and pelvic organ prolapse.
- A *colposcopist* – Ask them to take you through a colposcopy. Ask them how they describe CIN and how they explain to patients that excisional treatment is needed.
- A *sexual and reproductive health specialist* – Try and sit in a clinic and ask them to go through counselling and other pertinent issues relating to the termination of pregnancy and the management of sexually transmitted infections.

MENTAL AND PHYSICAL PREPARATION FOR THE MRCOG PART 3

We have used the word 'perform' a lot already in this book. That is because passing the MRCOG Part 3 exam requires a good performance. For written exams, preparing physically and psychologically is important. However, mental and physical preparation for the MRCOG Part 3 exam is even more important to optimise your performance.

Motivation

Stick to your realistic and achievable schedule. Once you have found out you have passed the MRCOG Part 2 exam, write your Part 3 preparation schedule and stick to it. This has benefits for your morale and motivation.

Allow time for relaxation

The MRCOG Part 3 exam can be immensely stressful to prepare for. Mainly, this comes from the fear of the unknown and needing to perform when an examiner is observing. What stations will come up? What if I cannot placate an angry patient? What if I go totally blank? The purpose of this book is to provide you with a strategy so that you have a method to deal with any of these eventualities. However, your levels of stress will inevitably be high as you are so close to obtaining your membership. It is therefore important to set some time to relax, exercise and spend time with your friends and family. This will allow you to put the importance of the exam into some perspective.

Exercise and diet

Your preparation will be much more effective if you can regularly exercise. Exercising allows you to clear your head and reduce stress levels as well as increases your focus when you sit down to revise again. Eating a healthy diet avoiding large, heavy meals will also improve your mental alertness.

Relaxation techniques

Utilising these techniques can be useful during the weeks before the exam as well as immediately prior to the Task Circuit when stress levels will be at their highest. Find a quiet place and take some deep breaths for 10 minutes. Visualising success is an important facet of executing a great performance so try and imagine doing well in stations. If meditation is not for you, listening to music or going for a walk is just as useful.

Strategic and mental planning

We have provided the strategies, techniques and approaches that you should take for each different type of task station. You may want to adopt these as we have suggested or change them slightly. Whatever you choose to do, you should have a well-defined strategy that you have used and practised multiple times before the actual day of the exam. This will enable you to be familiar with the technique that you will employ and to think a little deeper about each station. For example, you may choose to take a gynaecological history the way that we have suggested here, or you may choose to change the order that you ask questions slightly. Whichever method you use, it should be well practiced; you should not just make up the method on the day.

What if things go wrong?

It is almost inevitable that you will have at least one station that does not go well. You can reduce the chance of this happening with excellent preparation, but the feelings and emotions that you experience on the day of the exam will be unique. As scary as this may seem, you must try and imagine these events happening. Whether this is being shouted at for 10 minutes by an angry patient or going completely blank in a structured discussion task, you need to mentally prepare for these events so that you know how you will then deal with this difficult situation.

You should have prepared a strategy to deal with this situation, should it arise on the day of the exam. For example, in the situation of a 'mental blank', some candidates pause and ask the examiner for a few moments to collect their thoughts or to rephrase the question.

Importantly, remember that even if you perform poorly in one or two stations, you can still pass the exam. It is therefore essential for you to draw a line after each of the tasks, as the next examiner will not know that you have just had a terrible station. Prepare yourself for this before the day of the exam so it is not such a shock, should these events happen.

The night before and the morning of the exam

There is no point in cramming the night before the MRCOG Part 3 exam. This is more likely to be harmful to your performance than in any written exam. You must be sharp to perform well, and this means that you should stop working, relax, prepare your smart clothes and get enough sleep.

On the morning of the exam, get dressed early, have a light breakfast and have some brief notes to look at. Find yourself a quite space and use your relaxation techniques.

Practical arrangements

Be clear of the time and location of the exam. Plan your journey and accommodation. Do not risk rushing and adding to your stress levels. This should go without saying, but there are almost always candidates that arrive late for their Task Circuit!

SECTION II

TECHNIQUES FOR SPECIFIC OSCE STATIONS

CHAPTER 2
HISTORY AND
MANAGEMENT
STATIONS

The 'history and management' stations are a good opportunity for the clinically experienced candidate to shine. The majority of MRCOG Part 3 candidates will already have a few years of valuable clinical experience under their belts such that taking a relevant patient history, conducting an appropriate examination, arriving at a diagnosis and formulating a management plan are second nature. The ability to interact with the patient and to elicit important information represents some of the 'art' of medicine, whereas assimilating, interpreting and applying this received information represents more of the 'science' of medicine. As busy clinicians, you undertake this clinical process (Figure 2.1) implicitly in an often seamless fashion. In the context of the postgraduate clinical examination however, you need to display explicitly these fundamental clinical abilities to a third party. This requirement can sometimes throw the otherwise clinically competent candidate. Thus, as with all facets of the MRCOG Part 3 OSCE, an understanding of the station's requirements will allow suitable approaches to be developed and practised. Optimal performance requires preparation, even by the most clinically competent of candidates.

TAKING A PATIENT HISTORY

You all learnt the process of history taking as medical students and most of you will have had this generic skill observed and examined during your undergraduate years. As postgraduates, you are taught new practical skills, and your competency is assessed. The ability to take a history, however, is invariably 'taken as read' and consequently this most fundamental and crucial clinical skill is overlooked. From running clinical courses and examining MRCOG Part 3 candidates, it is surprising how many candidates perform poorly when asked to take and present a succinct clinical history. Nothing raises an examiner's 'antibodies' more than being forced to sit through a prolonged, largely irrelevant and convoluted history! (You can experience the feeling for yourself by asking a representative group of medical students to take and present histories to you.) In contrast, a confident, well taken, relevant and clearly presented history is a pleasure to witness and in practice the examiner may 'switch off' after the first minute as a result of the great first impression.

The main purpose of history taking is to aid the clinician in establishing a diagnosis (or certainly a list of diagnostic possibilities). It has been estimated that over 70% of diagnoses can be made on history alone. The main difference between a patient history taken by an undergraduate and a postgraduate is that the history

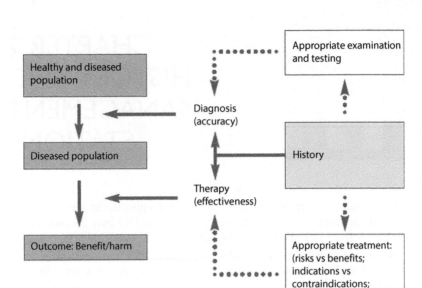

Figure 2.1 The clinical process.

has a 'purpose', i.e. it is the first and most important step in acquiring the clinical diagnosis so that appropriate treatments can be instituted. Medical students often consider treating a condition in an abstract way with little consideration for the patient or the need to develop appropriate management strategies. A good postgraduate candidate will display his/her clinical competence and maturity by taking these factors into account. In addition, a good interaction with the patient whilst obtaining a clinical history allows the doctor to develop a rapport with their patient, relate the history to the patient's health-related quality of life (HRQL), and direct the relevant physical examination, subsequent investigations and treatment. Try to convey empathy and confidence, thereby engendering a feeling of trust in your patients (and your examiner!) in your abilities.

In order to ensure a good performance, the following points should be considered and more importantly practised:

- **Preparation** – Read the question carefully and consider what the station is testing and what the likely diagnoses may be. Before entering the station, think about your introduction and opening few questions (a confident, enthusiastic, clear start ensures a good first impression and allows nerves to dissipate, improving subsequent performance).
- **Introduction** – Confident, clear and engage the patient (pleasant manner, eye contact, etc.).
- **Structure of history** – There are different approaches to obtaining a patient history. The aim is to obtain an efficient, comprehensive and relevant history in a logical sequence. The order of taking the history does not really matter as long as this aim is achieved. Standard structures for O&G histories are shown in the box nearby.

Standard structures for history taking in O&G

Obstetric history summary (template)

Mrs NAME is an AGE-year-old OCCUPATION presenting at NUMBER OF WEEKS' gestation in her NUMBER pregnancy with PRESENTING COMPLAINT (DURATION).

Additional sentence(s) – add any relevant risk factors, investigation results, diagnoses and management to date

Obstetric history
- Presenting complaint
- History of presenting complaint
- History of current pregnancy
- Past obstetric history
- Past medical history
- Drug history
- Family history
- Social history

Gynaecological history summary (template)

Mrs NAME is an AGE-year-old OCCUPATION presenting with PRESENTING COMPLAINT (DURATION). Additional sentence(s) – add any relevant risk factors, investigation results, diagnoses and management to date.

Gynaecological history
- Presenting complaint
- History of presenting complaint
- Systematic enquiry
- Past obstetric history
- Past medical history
- Drug history
- Family history
- Social history

Important points in the obstetric history

- **Context** – LMP (estimated date of delivery); gravidity + parity.
- **Presenting complaint (duration).**
- **History of presenting complaint:**
  Include onset, duration, progress, management, relevant symptoms and related risk factors for particular symptoms (this demonstrates to the examiner your understanding of potential diagnoses; important 'negative' answers are as important as positive responses).
  Foetal movements.
- **History of current pregnancy:**
  Pre-pregnancy (e.g. folic acid, rubella status, diabetic control); diagnosis of pregnancy; early pregnancy problems (bleeding, vomiting); gestation at booking; routine investigations (booking bloods, screening tests and scans).

Antenatal care to date (including plans of care, e.g. additional scans, day assessment unit appointments, glucose tolerance tests and emergency attendances/admissions).

- **Past obstetric history:**

  Chronological – Year of delivery and duration of pregnancy.

  Gravidity – Miscarriage/termination/ectopic – diagnosis and management.

  Parity – Onset of labour (induced or spontaneous); mode of delivery, reason for operative delivery, birth weight; gender; complications (antenatal, perinatal or postnatal); feeding.

- **Past medical history:**

  Identify important past or ongoing medical problems that may affect or be affected by the pregnancy.

  Consider also relevant past gynaecological history (infertility, last cervical smear and result).

  Past blood transfusion.

- **Drug history** – Indication; necessity; change of medication or dose in response to pregnancy; possible teratogenicity; allergies.

- **Family history** – Foetal anomalies; genetic conditions; consanguinity; diabetes; hypertension; pre-eclampsia; gestational diabetes; twins.

- **Social history** – Occupation; poor social circumstances; smoking; epidemiological risk factors for obstetric problems; misuse of prescribed/ recreational drugs.

Antenatal risk factors ('risk scoring')

- Poor obstetric history, e.g. preterm delivery, IUGR, foetal anomaly, stillbirth, abruption
- Extremes of age
- Extremes of weight
- Pre-existing medical conditions, e.g. diabetes, hypertension, psychiatric
- Significant family history
- Smokers
- Drug abusers
- Social deprivation
- Domestic violence

- **Presenting complaint** – main symptom(s) and duration.

- **History of presenting complaint:**

  Obtain information about the presenting complaint(s) including any tests/ treatments.

  Enquire further about other *relevant* gynaecological symptoms (this demonstrates your understanding of potential diagnoses to the examiner). Important 'negative' answers are as important as positive responses.

  Enquire routinely about cervical smear history and current contraception/ contraceptive history (and fertility plans, if appropriate) at the end of this part so as not to forget.

- **Systematic enquiry** – Cardiovascular; respiratory; gastrointestinal; musculoskeletal; central nervous system.
- **Obstetric history:**

  This can usually be brief for most gynaecological histories and restricted to number of pregnancies/children, mode of delivery and future fertility plans. However, more detailed exploration may be indicated in some circumstances, e.g. recurrent miscarriage, infertility, urogynaecology.
- **Past medical history:**

  Enquire about surgical history and past/current medical problems (often also a good time to ask about any medications for particular medical problems).

  Although 'unexpected' relevant past gynaecological history may arise, try to avoid this by enquiring about any relevant gynaecological history (diagnoses/tests/treatments) in the history of the presenting complaint.
- **Drug history** – Including allergies.
- **Family history** – Cancer, thrombophilia (if relevant).
- **Social history** – Occupation, marital status, tobacco, alcohol, recreational drugs/accommodation (if relevant).

Summary

You may be asked to present a succinct summary to the examiner. Indeed some candidates like to present this to the patient routinely at the end to clarify any issues and to confirm the validity of the history, i.e. the information obtained correctly reflects the patient's true history. This summary should contain the key points within two to three articulate sentences, which will influence further investigation and management. Avoid extraneous information, as the examiner will switch off! This can and should be rehearsed, e.g.

> Mrs X is a 48-year-old nulliparous hairdresser presenting with a 6-month history of non-cyclical pelvic pain that has been refractory to treatment with simple analgesics and the combined oral contraceptive pill. The pain is causing her to take time off work and is affecting her relationship with her family. She has been treated for presumed pelvic inflammatory disease in the past and a recent pelvic ultrasound has been reported as normal.

See further boxes nearby and Table 2.1.

Table 2.1 Features of good and bad history taking

Feature	Good history	Bad history
Interaction	Engages patient, listens	Disengaged, ignores answers
Questions	Open, unambiguous	Closed, ambiguous
Sequence	Logical, avoid repetition	Illogical, repetition
Emphasis	Focused on presenting complaint	'Scattergun', vague
Information	Relevant, facilitates differential diagnoses	Irrelevant, inability to arrive at differential diagnoses
Time to acquire	Rapid	Slow
Presentation	Succinct, germane	Drawn out, extraneous information

Revision checklist for gynaecological histories of presenting complaint

- **Menstrual:**

  LMP, amount, regularity, duration of menses/cycle length, impact on HRQL, dysmenorrhoea and timing/duration, IMB, PCB, age of menarche, perimenopausal symptoms (as appropriate), symptoms of anaemia.

  Primary vs secondary amenorrhoea, oligomenorrhoea, menopausal symptoms, weight change, acne, seborrhoea, hirsutism, galactorrhoea.

- **Chronic pelvic pain** – Site, onset, character, radiation, periodicity (particularly in relation to the menstrual cycle), duration, relieving/exacerbating factors, associated symptoms, dyspareunia (deep/superficial), GIT/GU systemic enquiry.

- **Vaginal discharge** – Colour, odour, amount, itch, cyclical, past history of sexually transmitted infection, diabetes.

- **Urogynaecological** – Frequency, volume of voids, thirst, fluid intake, urgency, inability to interrupt flow, dysuria, strangury, haematuria, nocturia, incontinence (stress and provoking factors, urge), prolapse (vaginal discomfort, back pain; feeling of something coming down), bowel function.

- **Fertility:**

  Female – Menstrual, reproductive/sexual history (frequency of coitus, libido, dyspareunia), past obstetric history, past medical history (especially history of sexually transmitted infections/abdominal sepsis/ tubal surgery).

  Male – Reproductive/sexual history (impotence, ejaculation), past medical history (especially history of sexually transmitted infections/genital operations), social history (environmental and/or occupational exposure to hazardous factors, e.g. smoking, alcohol; occupation (sedentary)).

- **Premenstrual syndrome** – cyclical physical and mental symptoms, headaches, bloating, breast tenderness, change in mood, irritability.

- **Menopausal** – hot flushes, night sweats and insomnia, mood alteration, vaginal dryness, lack of libido, fatigue.

Top tips for patient history taking

1. Ask open-ended questions rather than leading ones and do not use medical terms, e.g. do you have menorrhagia? To speed the history along in a systematic fashion you will probably need to ask more closed, targeted questions to obtain a more detailed description of symptoms in order to formulate a logical history in a coherent fashion. The art is to demonstrate to the examiner that you are giving the patient time to describe in her own words what she perceives to be the problem(s) but are keeping the sequence of questions and responses 'on track'.

2. In a typical obstetric or gynaecological history, it is unlikely that a detailed social history (in contrast to elderly care medicine/psychiatry) or drug history/systematic enquiry (unlike general medical histories) will be required but be prepared for this, e.g. domestic violence/drug abuse in an antenatal patient.

3. Concentrate upon the *history of the presenting complaint* and related history rather than trying to be totally 'comprehensive' – trying to cover all aspects of a history leads to loss of focus and confusion, i.e. you end up not being able to 'see the wood for the trees'. This does not mean overlooking other aspects of the history (see above) as these can be taken quite quickly and will gain you marks on the examiner's structured mark sheet. However, discretionary marks and overall marks will be optimised by staying focused upon the *history of the presenting complaint*, thereby producing an individual, tailored history and understanding the fact that a detailed 'micro-history' of every known obstetric or gynaecological symptom is not required.

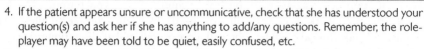

4. If the patient appears unsure or uncommunicative, check that she has understood your question(s) and ask her if she has anything to add/any questions. Remember, the role-player may have been told to be quiet, easily confused, etc.
5. Be aware of the requirements of good history taking (see Table 2.1) so you leave the examiner with a favourable impression of your performance.

MANAGEMENT

As practising O&G, you spend a large part of your working week formulating what you hope are the most effective, appropriate and acceptable management plans for your patients. It should come as no surprise, therefore, that the MRCOG Part 3 clinical examination will seek to assess your competency in this important area. Such stations will ask you to *outline* or *discuss* or *explain* a *plan of management* or perhaps *management options* with your patient.

The fact you have been invited to attend the clinical examination means that you have already demonstrated to the satisfaction of the RCOG your clinical knowledge *on paper*. The key now is to demonstrate that this knowledge can be put into practice in the 'real' clinical environment. In the written paper, you are conveying your knowledge to the examiner reading your manuscript. Although you may be asked direct set questions regarding clinical management (a structured 'viva') in the practical OSCE, it is more common that you will need to convey your knowledge to the examiner via your interaction with the 'patient' sitting in front of you. Clearly this sort of station does not just test your ability to devise an appropriate management strategy (often based upon your preceding history); it also tests your skill in communication (see Chapter 3).

Tips on how to approach these two types of clinical management stations are outlined below.

Discuss management with examiner: structured viva

In general, the examiner will ask questions around the management of O&G problems presenting in an elective (e.g. clinic, inpatient ward, operating theatre) or emergency setting (e.g. labour ward, acute gynaecology unit, A&E department). Make sure you listen carefully to the questions posed and do not rush into an answer without due consideration. It is likely that you have dealt with a similar clinical problem either directly or indirectly and so use this experience to aid you when responding. It is usually quite apparent to the examiner as to which candidates have experience of managing such clinical problems and which need to rely heavily on theoretical 'textbook' recollection of facts.

The beauty of clinical medicine is its diversity and so it is naïve to think that there is always a clear 'right' or 'wrong' answer to managing specific clinical problems. The clinically mature candidate will be able to convey this complexity by considering more than one approach to management whilst avoiding appearing indecisive. A good way of doing this is to outline the available management options, succinctly summarise the pros and cons of each intervention but then come down on what *you would actually do*.

Even if the examiner disagrees with you or your chosen option is not the one advocated on the structured mark sheet, you will score marks by having considered alternative options, and your clinical consideration will score overall 'global' discretionary marks. Two examples of this approach are given in the boxes nearby.

Example 1: Approach to discussing management options

Would you agree to undertake a hysterectomy in a fit 51-year-old perimenopausal woman with menorrhagia and uterine fibroids who is requesting this intervention despite a benign endometrial biopsy and not having received any medical treatment for the symptom prior to referral?

Consider:

- **Pros vs cons:**
  Pros – Effective treatment; medical treatments more likely to fall in the presence of uterine fibroids; surgical morbidity is likely to be low in an otherwise fit patient.
  Cons – Natural menopause imminent; patient may respond well to medical or minimally invasive surgical options; higher surgical morbidity with hysterectomy.
- **Patient preferences** – Impact on her HRQL; understanding and awareness of less invasive treatment options and menopause.

Answer – Despite the fact that her bleeding symptoms are likely to resolve soon naturally, in the presence of uterine pathology, I would agree to her request if her symptoms are having a significant adverse impact on her HRQL and she understands the risks associated with surgery and that other effective, simpler treatment options are available.

Example 2: Approach to discussing management options

Would you induce a woman at 36 weeks with an unfavourable cervix who is complaining of pelvic discomfort and difficulty mobilising attributed to symphysis pubis dysfunction? She has had one previous pregnancy that resulted in an elective caesarean section for a breech presentation and she would like a trial of vaginal delivery this time.

Consider:

- **Pros vs cons:**
  Pros – SPD may improve more quickly and improve HRQL.
  Cons – Increased likelihood of failed IOL and emergency C/S in labour (resulting in longer post-delivery convalescence and prolonged mobility limitations); need for IOL on labour ward as high risk; small risk RDS in preterm neonate; no evidence for benefit of early IOL (or C/S).
- **Patient preferences** – Impact on her HRQL; understanding and awareness of SPD and the potential risks and benefits; conservative treatment options (positional advice; analgesics, physiotherapy, belts).

Answer – Given the facts she has not laboured before, is preterm and has an unfavourable cervix and a uterine scar, on balance quicker resolution of her symptoms (especially if she ends up with an emergency C/S) cannot be guaranteed with induction. I would not advise IOL, but would try to persuade her to delay IOL until at least around 38 weeks if her cervix becomes more favourable. I would explain to her that I believe the risks outweigh any potential benefit, whilst recognising the impact her symptoms are having on her HRQL, and so would aim to optimise management (analgesics, physiotherapy) and offer her weekly follow-up and additional midwifery support.

Discuss management with patient (role-player)

At this situation, you must concentrate on the patient, establish a rapport with her and ignore the presence of the examiner. If the station has instructed you to discuss management, i.e. *not* to take a preceding history, then remember to introduce yourself. At all times, however difficult the interaction may become, remain composed and appear professional. Remember that the consultation may not be going well either because you are not communicating well or the role- player has been instructed to be uncommunicative or difficult, i.e. she has a set agenda. If the patient is quiet, you should probe for a response by checking if she has understood or has any questions or concerns, requires clarification or has any specific preferences for treatment. Listen and do not interrupt or talk over the patient unless she is being unduly verbose (which she may have been instructed to be!). Whilst you want to convey to the examiner your ability to address all viable management options, you must avoid giving too much information to the patient without pausing for a response from the patient – give information in small 'chunks'. Some candidates like to draw diagrams to aid explanation and patient understanding, but unless this is something you employ in your day-to-day practice (and are good at!), then trying such an approach for the first time in an exam situation may be counterproductive.

Summary of approach to management stations involving a role-player

- Introduce yourself.
- Explain why you are there.
- Remain composed and in control of the consultation – be aware that the role-player may have been briefed to be difficult.
- Avoid talking too much and concentrate on communication:
  Break up the consultation by providing information in small 'chunks'.
  Ask if she has any questions, concerns, preferences or needs you to explain again/ provide clarification.
  Use diagrams only if this is part of your usual practice.
- Do not interact with the examiner unless instructed to do so.

EXAMPLE QUESTION

Candidate's instructions

This station is a role-play station and will assess your abilities to take a concise and relevant history; address the patient's anxiety and outline the treatment options available. You will be assessed using the following domains:

- Patient safety
- Communication with patients and their relatives
- Information gathering
- Applied clinical knowledge

The patient you are about to see is Cindy Ray, a 23-year-old law student who has been referred because of severe period pain. Her GP found no abnormality on examination but she has been told that she may have something called 'adenomyosis' which has made her very anxious.

Simulated role-player's instructions

You are Cindy Ray, a 23-year-old law student. You are single and have never been sexually active. You have no medical problems of note but smoke 20 cigarettes a day and drink socially.

Your menstrual cycles are regular and not heavy but are very painful. The pain is colicky, suprapubic and starts 2 days before your period and generally eases off around day 3 of your period. You have suffered with this pain since menarche aged 16 years. The pain can be so severe as to leave you bed-bound so that you take time off from your studies. You take co-codamol on an ad hoc basis to combat the pain, but you do not like taking tablets. You do not have any other pain and minimal PMS symptoms.

You are anxious because you have been told you have a disease called adenomyosis, a condition that you do not fully understand but you have read that the condition necessitates a hysterectomy.

Marking

Patient safety

- Takes a comprehensive history in order to offer safe therapeutic options in the management plan.
- Suggests appropriate and safe therapeutic options for the management of chronic pelvic pain.

Communication with patients and their relatives

- Demonstrates good communication skills during history taking.
- Acknowledges the patient's concerns and anxieties.
- Explains the treatment options available in a logical manner.
- Adopts a mutualistic form of consultation to produce a clear management plan to tackle the patient's chronic pelvic pain.

Information gathering

- Demonstrates a clear structure when taking a gynaecological history.
- Takes all of the details required for a comprehensive history.
- Listens to the patient attentively and allows good flow of information.
- Assesses the wish of the patient regarding their preferred therapeutic options.

Applied clinical knowledge

- Evidence that the candidate attempts to deduce the most likely diagnosis from the history taken and the questions asked.

- Understands the medical and surgical options available in patients with chronic pelvic pain.
- Demonstrates knowledge of the paramedical therapies available in chronic pelvic pain.

Examiner's instructions

In this station, the candidate should be able to take an appropriate history whilst also ascertain the reasons for the patient's anxiety. The candidate should be able to address anxiety and discuss the possible diagnoses and the appropriate management options.

The nature, site, pattern (in relation to menstrual cycle) and duration of pain, precipitating/relieving factors, previous treatment, menstrual bleeding history, previous obstetric history, contraceptive/sexual history and relevant medical problems should be ascertained

The candidate should be able to ascertain the reasons for her anxiety, which include the following:

- Labelled as having a disease 'adenomyosis' at a young age.
- Uncertainty about the condition and its implications.
- Fear of needing a hysterectomy and its effect on femininity/fertility.

The candidate should then address the reasons for her anxiety and then explain the possible diagnoses:

- Explanation of diagnosis 'spasmodic primary dysmenorrhoea'.
- Explanation of adenomyosis in simple lay terms and its implications (minimal, can be associated with endometriosis). *Adenomyosis is a common condition in which tissue that normally lines the uterus (the endometrium) begins to grow inside the muscular outer wall of the uterus which can lead to heavy menstrual bleeding, pain and sometimes an enlargement of the uterus.*
- **General context** – Spasmodic dysmenorrhoea commoner in nulliparous (young) women (up to 50%), most of whom do not have adenomyosis. May improve after childbirth. Whether adenomyosis or not is irrelevant, as it is the *symptoms* that are treated. Diagnosis is histological (at hysterectomy) but treatment does not necessitate a hysterectomy unless the patient is an older woman without future fertility aspirations and who is refractory to other less invasive therapies.
- **Individual context** – Adenomyosis unlikely from symptoms as primary rather than secondary dysmenorrhoea, i.e. relieved with menstrual flow, no pain at other times of cycle (endometriosis, which is associated with adenomyosis, is unlikely). Classically, expect heavy periods and enlarged uterus which she does not have.

Appropriate management options should be discussed.

- Transabdominal ultrasound (note VI so not transvaginal) may help provide reassurance regarding pelvic anatomy/absence of gynaecological pathology and specifically adenomyosis (although scan has limited accuracy, as does MRI, but if uterus is of normal size and non-suggestive myometrial appearances, then adenomyosis is unlikely).

- General – Reassurance, general lifestyle – diet (healthy, oily fish, reduce dairy), exercise, stop smoking. Topical heat (about 39°C).
- Vitamins – B_1 and E – 2 days before, first 3 days of menses (RCT suggests benefit, Grade A evidence).
- Simple analgesics – Recommend NSAIDs, e.g. mefanamic acid – encourage taking these regularly rather than ad hoc for better pain control and use paracetamol or codeine in between doses. If patient does not like taking tablets, consider rectal suppositories or transdermal preparations.
- First-line hormonal manipulation – COC, try sequential at first, then consider tricycle or continuous.
- Second-line hormonal manipulation – Long-acting progestogens (DMPA, Implanon, Mirena).
- Other – Transcutaneous electrical nerve stimulation (high frequency stimulation).
- Surgical – Third-line, definitive evidence from large RCT that laparoscopic uterosacral nerve ablation is not effective; no strong evidence of benefit and potential for significant morbidity with laparoscopic presacral neurectomy.

CHAPTER 3
COMMUNICATION, COUNSELLING AND BREAKING BAD NEWS

Since the introduction of the clinical OSCE to MRCOG Part 3 examination with its use of professional role-players, it is fair to say that the 'communication and counselling' stations have instilled fear and loathing in equal measure in the prospective part 3 candidate. Candidates recount in vivid detail their traumatic experiences with grief stricken 'patients' or, worse still, encounters with hot-headed 'relatives', apparently incandescent with rage. Although these accounts can shake the most confident candidate, the truth is that with adequate preparation and a modicum of knowledge, these stations can not only be successfully navigated but can be a fruitful source of easy marks. Hopefully, by the end of this chapter, you will no longer approach these stations with trepidation but embrace them.

APPROACH TO THE STATION

It is possible for the 'bookworm' to pass the written part of the MRCOG Part 3 exam with limited actual clinical time 'spent at the coalface'. However, the clinical OSCE is designed to assess a candidate's clinical experience and so validate their competence to proceed in a career in O&G. OSCE stations requiring 'communication or counselling' are exemplary for assessing competence in dealing with 'real life situations', which cannot simply be 'learnt' from a textbook. In view of this, you should concentrate upon showing your counselling skills and not be preoccupied with conveying your knowledge of a subject area. The latter is *not* what is required. You have passed the written part of the MRCOG examination and so your knowledge is taken as read.

That said, there are undoubtedly techniques and approaches to counselling stations that can be practised and 'learnt'. This chapter deals with both generic and specific approaches to communication and counselling situations you may encounter in the exam.

General approach to communications and counselling stations

Recognise the paramount importance of your introduction and manner

- Greet, introduce, gain permission, eye contact.
- Speak in a calm and purposeful manner.
- Explain why you are here.
- Listen attentively.

- Sympathetic approach – Express condolences, recognise her tragic loss, respect her views.
- Do not appear rushed or defensive.
- Be honest and do not hesitate to admit what you do not know because maintaining trust matters more than appearing knowledgeable.
- Establish a relationship with the patient.

Recognise the importance of supportive nonverbal communication

- Maintaining eye contact
- Nodding
- Smiling
- Looks of concern
- Tactile, if appropriate

Allow patients to express grief/anger

- Do not 'jump in', i.e. listen attentively and do not interrupt, so allowing patients to disclose their feelings, worries and concerns.
- Allow silences/pauses.
- Offer to come back again if she would like time to herself.
- Encourage the patient/family to speak honestly.
- Display empathy (verbal and nonverbal) – let the woman know that she is being listened to and understood with non-verbal prompts and verbal 'paraphrasing' of what has been said by them (*Examples*: 'I can see how angry you are about what happened'; 'So you feel very annoyed that no one explained the situation to you…'; 'It must be hard for you with…').
- Recognise the need to address/acknowledge/validate the emotion expressed (*Examples*: 'This must be difficult for you. Can you tell me how you are feeling?' or 'I can see that you are angry'.).
- Repeat/reinforce information several times and 'offer' to give written information, if possible to back up.

GENERAL COMMUNICATION TECHNIQUES AND SKILLS

Provision of effective and compassionate care requires a good doctor–patient relationship. Such a relationship relies greatly on effective communication. A combination of evidence and theory shows that good communication can improve accuracy of diagnosis, compliance with treatment, clinical outcomes (such as blood pressure and blood glucose levels), a patient's trust in the clinician, patient satisfaction and, last but not least, the clinician's satisfaction. It can also reduce the risk of litigation.

The ability to assess communication skills is the primary advantage an OSCE offers compared to the written MRCOG exam. Effective communication has several components; many of us do most of these naturally. However, careful consideration of the various facets of communication is likely to improve its effectiveness and, of course, enhance the chances of passing the exam! Research evidence has now rejected the traditional opinion that good communication skills are something intrinsic, and little can be done if you are not gifted with such skills. Studies, both within and outside medicine, show that communications skills can be taught, learnt and examined. We provide some didactic guidelines in this chapter.

Greet

You don't get a second chance to make the first impression.

(Anonymous)

Let's let the evidence speak. A study of 415 patients showed that 91% of them wanted the doctor to address them by name, with 50% preferring the forename, 17% the surname and the rest both names. The same survey found that only 50% of doctors observed this basic expectation of their patients. On the much discussed 'to shake or not to shake' debate, 78% of patients showed a preference to shake hands with their doctor.

So, our evidence-based recommendation is for you to greet the patient with their name ('Good morning, Mrs Smith'), introduce yourself ('I am Dr Patel'), and offer to shake hands unless you or the patient may be averse to this for cultural or other reasons. Using the patient's forename and surname in an initial greeting will not only set the scene for a good doctor–patient relationship but also ensure correct identification of patients, which is an elemental aspect of patient safety.

Names are not just for greeting. Use of a patient's name through the consultation gives her the reassurance that you see her as an individual, and not merely as the next 'case' on the clinic conveyor belt. How much better it is to say, 'Mrs Smith, can you please tell me about any past operations?' than 'Next, can you please tell me about any past operations?' Of course, every sentence need not start with the patient's name, but occasional use of her name will add a personal touch.

Define the purpose of the encounter

No meeting should start without an agenda. A medical consultation is no different. Simple explanation of the purpose is likely to put the patient at ease, and give you and the patient a common point to start from. For example, you may start with, 'Your GP has written telling me that you have heavy periods. Is that your main complaint?' If the patient confirms, then you may go on to set out a joint agenda for the consultation: 'I would like to obtain details of your symptoms, perform an examination, arrange any necessary tests, and discuss possible management options. Are you happy with this plan?' Such a roadmap is essential to make sure both you and your patient do not get lost during the consultation.

However, very few patients come to a doctor with a single problem. Besides, the reason for referral could have changed. For example, a GP may have referred a patient with heavy periods, but since then an ultrasound arranged to investigate the heavy periods could have shown a large ovarian cyst, which might now be the patient's main complaint. Simply 'letting the patient talk' will elicit such issues. Once you have elicited all the main complaints, negotiate and prioritise the agenda.

Let the patient talk

Research evidence shows that doctors allow patients only 23 seconds to present their story before interrupting! Only 2% of patients feel they get the opportunity to complete their story. This is likely to result in severe restriction of flow of information from the patient, which in turn can compromise the diagnostic process and patient satisfaction. It can also lead to the fateful exam situation in which the OSCE role-player asks you, 'What about the 10 cm ovarian cyst that my GP was concerned about?', in the final minute of the OSCE station when you are busy rapidly regurgitating treatment options for menorrhagia!

Our recommendation is for you to ask the patient, 'Tell me what is troubling you', and then to sit back and listen until she is ready to stop. In the OSCE situation, aim to give the patient at least 90 seconds – research shows that a patient's average opening statement (if uninterrupted) is shorter than 90 seconds. Occasionally, a patient may start to throw a number of seemingly unrelated issues at you (my heavy periods, hair loss and right little toe are troubling me). In that situation, it is reasonable to suggest that the patient focuses on one issue at a time, with a promise that you will hear out the others later: 'Tell me about your periods first; you can tell me about the other problems later.

Top tip!

All candidates 'talk too much'. Therefore, consciously concentrate upon allowing pauses and not 'jumping in'. This approach will allow the patient/relative to express their concerns. Remember that the role-player has a scenario and mark sheet to follow, and the adoption of such a strategy is likely to give you valuable information and elicit clues as to where the station is leading and where the marks are to be collected.

Listen

Listening is a learnable skill, although a tough one to master. The four elements of good listening are as follows:

- Paying attention
- Not interrupting
- Echoing
- Appropriate nonverbal language

Let's take these in turn. 'Paying attention' refers to listening with a genuine interest and registering in your mind (and the notes) what the patient has to say; those doctors who have no interest in doing this are probably in the wrong profession. You should switch off your phone, clear your mind of other raging thoughts and get into the frame of mind of: 'I am here to listen to you and help you'. The patient should feel there is no urgency and she has your undivided attention.

'Not interrupting' does not refer to deathly silences which can be discomforting to most patients. It does, however, mean not butting in with questions like, 'How many pads?', 'Any clots?' Encouraging the patient to go on with expressions such as 'Uh-huh', 'I see', 'Yes' and 'Go on' can, of course, be employed.

Echoing refers to the technique that encourages patient to talk and shows empathy.

Example of echoing

Mrs Smith: The periods are now out of control, doctor. None of the medicines seems to work. I use tampons and towels and am still getting blood dripping down my legs. I am so fed up with it…

Doctor: Uh-huh.

Mrs Smith: … and I have to take 3–4 days off work every month. My employer is fed up with me and I am fed up with my periods.

Doctor: Both you and your employer are fed up with the situation. (**echoing**)

Mrs Smith: Exactly! And my doctor doesn't seem to take it seriously either. I am popping so many tablets, but what good has that done to me?

Doctor: Yes, I see… nothing seems to work…. (**echoing**)

Mrs Smith: Well yes, more or less. The pill did work though for a while, but I didn't want to carry on taking it after my mum died of a dot in the chest…

Finally, appropriate nonverbal language is the hallmark of good listening skills. Appropriate eye contact, body posture (e.g. arms uncrossed and upper body slightly leaning forward) and use of nods and grunts all let the patient know that you are listening. Remember, it has been said 'nonverbal language speaks louder than verbal language', and if there is discordance between your verbal and nonverbal language, the patient will always believe your nonverbal message.

Question and discuss

The need to let the patient talk and listening must be balanced against your need to obtain a systematic history that allows you to examine various hypotheses regarding potential diagnosis and therapy. After the first 1 or 2 minutes, after the patient has had a chance to tell you her story, you will generally need to guide, quiz, redirect and focus on certain aspects of the story to complete the history. You will need to employ a combination of open ('Tell me about your periods?') and closed questions ('How many days do you bleed for?').

Example of good questioning (continued from the previous scenario)

Mrs Smith: Well yes, more or less. The pill did work though for a while, but I didn't want to carry on taking it after my mum died of a dot in the chest...I didn't want to die like her... and now this ovarian cyst...I feel my body is falling apart... and I am only 27.

Doctor: Mrs Smith, I think I understand what brought you here today. Three issues: your heavy periods, the ovarian cyst and concern about whether what happened to your mother could happen to you. (**echoing**) Shall we discuss your periods first? How long have they been a problem? (**focusing**)

Mrs Smith: For a good while, doctor.

Doctor: How long might that be in months and years? (**guiding**)

Mrs Smith: Oh... I don't know... maybe 2 years... maybe 3.

Doctor: OK, I see. You haven't kept an accurate record of it, but it sounds like it has been a problem for 2–3 years.

Mrs Smith: Yes. And the cyst was diagnosed 2 months ago, and I have got some heaviness on the right side and I think it could be due to the cyst.

Doctor: Yes, the heaviness could be related to the cyst. I can see the cyst is worrying you, and we will come back to that and discuss it in detail. However, before we go on to that, shall we finish our discussion on your periods. Tell me please, Mrs Smith, how many days do you bleed for when you have your periods? (**redirecting**)

Provide information and share decision-making

Patient's concerns usually revolve around one of two broad issues:

- Apprehension about the condition (diagnosis, prognosis and cause)
- Anxiety about the medical care (tests and treatment)

Research shows clinicians spend very little time, in some studies just 1 minute, providing information on the illness and options for treatment. An uninformative (from the *patient's view*) consultation can result in a patient visiting her GP seeking further information, non-compliance with tests and treatment, non-attendance at clinics and poor outcome. A robust way to provide information and share decision-making is to use the 'educational sandwich' of ATA – Ask, Tell and Ask.

The first 'Ask' relates to the clinician finding out what the patient's ideas, thoughts and feelings are about the cause, diagnosis, prognosis and treatment of the condition. This step is uniformly ignored by doctors, probably due to its perceived irrelevance. ('With my medical education and MRCOG, I know a great deal about this condition – what would this patient know other than half-truths, misconceptions? Why waste my time exploring these, when I can usefully provide a lecture on this condition?') When planning a route on a map, you need to know the starting location and the destination – if you have no idea of where you are on the map, there is no hope of planning a route to your destination. The same is true with the provision of medical information. Unless you know where your patient 'is' at the outset, your efforts to provide information will not get you very far. How do you put the first 'Ask' of ATA into practice? This is illustrated in the example in the box nearby.

Example of asking patient for her views about her condition (first 'ask' of ATA)

Doctor: Mrs Smith, before I explain the ovarian cyst, it would help me to know what you have already learnt about this and what your concerns are. (An alternative is: 'Mrs Smith, people normally have some ideas about ovarian cysts. What are your thoughts?') **(First 'Ask' of ATA)**

Mrs Smith: Well, yes, doctor, I know what you are going to say [*tears rolling down the face*]. My aunt had the same. I was fearing the worst.

Doctor [offering tissues, and leaning forward with concern]: I am sorry to see you upset, Mrs Smith. You mentioned fearing the worst?

Mrs Smith: Cancer, doctor, what else?

Doctor: That's a frightening thought. I see why you are troubled. Mrs Smith, please don't be troubled. You do not have cancer. What you have is what we call a 'simple cyst'; many women of your age have such cysts. It is a benign condition. We will of course do a blood test to be on the safe side. Of course, if it is causing you pain and you are terribly concerned, we also have the option of removing it.

Mrs Smith: Thank heavens, doctor. I haven't slept for days worrying about this. I didn't even tell my husband as I didn't want to worry him. Oh, my poor children, I have been so worried for them.

Doctor: I am glad I was able to help you with this, Mrs Smith. Now, let me turn to…

Whilst cancer was certainly not at the top of the doctor's differential list of items to discuss, it was right at the top of the patient's agenda. If the doctor had not specifically elicited the patient's views about her condition, she may have withheld from sharing it (as was the case with her husband) and the doctor's lectures about CA-125, laparoscopic drainage versus cystectomy, potential complications of laparoscopy, etc. would have fallen on deaf ears. Always remember that not all patients are forthcoming with questions and concerns – it is your job to probe if your desire is to help the patient.

The second step of ATA is to tell. Use a variety of approaches. Do not use medical jargon; if you must use jargon, then define it. Describe the condition or treatment in words, rephrase your description if it is a particularly complex concept, draw diagrams, use pictures and models, provide written information, use DVDs and, if there is a good information website, direct the patient to it. Clearly, many of these approaches cannot be taken in the OSCE exam, but there is nothing to stop you from drawing a sketch of the gynaecological organs to help the patient (the role-player) understand the information you wish to impart. You will generally need to cover the following three broad issues:

- What has happened to me? Is it serious? **(diagnosis and prognosis)**

- Why? (**causation**)
- What will be done to me? And when? (**tests and therapy**)

The final A of ATA refers to asking the patient again to describe what she understands. Understanding relies on transmission (from the doctor), reception (by the patient) and clarification (by both parties). The pragmatic way to assess if the patient has understood is to ask her to summarise the discussion. Two approaches are commonly recommended for this purpose, as illustrated in the box nearby.

Example of asking patient to summarise a discussion (final A of ATA sandwich)

Approach 1

Doctor: When you go home, your husband will probably ask you about the discussions we have had today. Please tell me what you will tell him? This will help me understand if I have explained the various issues sufficiently.

Approach 2

Doctor: I would like to make sure I have explained the issues clearly. Please tell me what you heard so that I can check to see if I have explained the issues adequately.

A simple 'is it OK?' is simply not OK. The questions, 'Is there anything else you would like me to tell you?' and 'Is there any aspect you would like me to go over again?', should complement the approaches above and not replace them!

At the completion of the visit, the clinician can summarise the agreed plans and discuss the next steps (next appointment, referral for tests or therapy elsewhere). There is a view held by some experts that patients regress into a state of juvenile dependence, hoping that the doctor will know what's wrong with them, perhaps with the help of some tests; furthermore, there is the view that there is a single best treatment for most conditions. This, unfortunately, is the exception in medicine. Good communication skills are essential in bridging the many gaps between clinicians and patients, and patients' stories and clinician's history records, so that good quality care can be provided.

Summary of general approach to communication and counselling stations

- Greet.
- Define the purpose of the encounter.
- Let the patient talk.
- Listen.
- Question and discuss.
- Provide information and share decision-making.

DIFFICULT COMMUNICATION SITUATIONS

Certain situations can be difficult for the patient, doctor or both. However, there are often tried and tested approaches that can be used to enhance the outcomes in such situations. In this section, we take you through the most important ones and provide practical help, including phrases and sentences you can use to help your patient, help yourself and, of course, help you pass your OSCE exam! You need to have primed yourself with the contents of Chapter 2 and Section "General Communication Techniques and Skills" to get the most out of this section.

GIVING BAD NEWS

Breaking bad news is difficult, and as a clinician you have to develop skills to connect and communicate effectively with your patients. Bad news and tragic outcomes can be very disturbing for all concerned and evoke a range of emotions. It is acceptable to empathise with someone's difficult situation, sadness, shock, tragedy, loss. Remember that this is a professional examination and these stations are an opportunity for the RCOG to assess your competence in dealing with 'real-life situations' which cannot be 'learnt' from a textbook. We recommend the following steps for 'good' delivery of bad news.

STEP 1: PREPARE

Preparation is the key. In your OSCE, take your time to *read and understand* the information provided on the station notice board and prepare your approach before entering the exam cubicle and facing the patient (the role-player). In real practice, pore over the notes, discuss the case with your senior colleagues, nurses and other relevant professionals and find out as much as possible about the condition (particularly, prognosis, therapy and support) before meeting the patient. Choose a quiet place where you are unlikely to be interrupted. Turn your phone off. Decide whether you wish to have a nurse or another person present.

STEP 2: GIVE A WARNING NOTE (OR TWO)

A patient needs to be ready to receive the bad news. For example, the following discourse is unlikely to register fully in the mind of a patient: 'Good Morning, Mrs Taylor. I am afraid the ultrasound shows the baby has passed away'. This is referred to as 'dropping the bomb' – warning notes avoid this situation. We show how warning notes are used in two different situations to prepare the patient.

Example of giving warning notes

Situation 1

You are the senior registrar and an experienced obstetric scanner. You have been called in to see a term woman after your registrar has been unable to find the foetal heart on ultrasound. Your scanning shows the absence of a foetal heart – the diagnosis is stillbirth.

Doctor: Mrs Taylor, I am unable to see any movements of the baby on the scan. (**warning note 1**)

Doctor: … and I am unable to see the baby's heartbeat. (**warning note 2**)

Mrs Taylor: Oh my God, Oh my God, is the baby dead?

Doctor: I am really sorry to give you this news… Yes, the baby has died.

Situation 2

You are about to give the information that an endometrial biopsy from a woman with PMB has shown endometrial cancer.

Doctor: Mrs Davis, I would like to discuss the findings of the biopsy you had last week, if that is OK with you.

Mrs Davis: Go right ahead doctor, I have been anxious to find out. Was it a polyp?

Doctor: We were hoping it would be just a polyp… but I am afraid the news is worse than that. (**warning note 1**)

Doctor: Some of the cells looked abnormal under the microscope. (**warning note 2**)

Mrs Davis: Abnormal?

Doctor: Yes, the biopsy shows it is in fact cancer of the lining of the womb.

Mrs David: You said it is cancer?

Doctor: Yes, it is cancer. (**repetition**)

Mrs Davis: Oh my God, I am going to die.

Doctor: Is that how it sounds… like it is all over… there is no hope? (**echoing**)

Patient: What can I hope with cancer?

Doctor: Well, many people with cancer can be successfully treated. People have different understanding of the word cancer. Can you please bear to tell me what it means to you? (**First 'Ask' for ATA**, see above)

(Once the doctor has established an understanding of Mrs Davis' ideas, concerns and expectations (ICE) regarding cancer and cancer treatment, they are in a position to provide effective counselling.)

STEP 3: PLAY IT STRAIGHT

Once the warning note(s) has been given, the patient will not only be ready, but also very likely anxious, to know the finding. After giving the warning note(s), it is cruel to meander around the issue with trivialities such as 'Did you find parking OK?' or 'The weather is changing fast, isn't it?' or even with relevant but perhaps less pressing issues such as 'Tell me, how is the pain now?' or 'Do you have anyone to look after you at home?' The rule is that after the warning note, the bad news needs to be given. It is important to use non-technical language (e.g. cancer not neoplasm) and to be honest (cancer and not 'a bit of a growth'). Whilst it is important to break the bad news with appropriate affect, there is no need to go into 'undertaker mode' with exaggerated gloominess and hopelessness.

STEP 4: BE RESPONSIVE AND REPEAT AS OFTEN AS NECESSARY

As receiving bad news can often induce a degree of temporary mental paralysis, be ready to find out how much has been absorbed by patient and what would be usefully repeated by you. You have to tell a little, pause, observe the reaction and tell a little bit more or repeat as necessary. You may want to provide written information and must always leave the patient with an avenue to get support (from you, the team or an emergency telephone line).

STEP 5: GIVE (APPROPRIATE) HOPE

Even in the bleakest situations, there are reasons for hope. For example, someone with a terminal cancer may find hope in the possibility of a period of remission or the prospect of a pain-free peaceful death. Never get into the game of giving precise prognostications about survival – whatever you say is likely to be wrong! An approach to handling a survival question is illustrated in the box nearby.

Example of handling a survival question

Mrs Davis has terminal cancer. You have offered palliative care.

Mrs Davis: Doctor, how long have I got?

Doctor: Mrs Davis, I am sorry. The trouble is none of us knows. It depends on how you respond to the treatment and many other issues.

Mrs Davis: Doctor, will I be here for Christmas?

Doctor: I realise the uncertainly must be terrible for you. Mrs Davis, I am really sorry, but there is no way of predicting the future. However, what I can do is to put forward the symptoms and signs that you could look for to see if you are deteriorating. Would it help if I told you what they are?

Mrs Davis: Yes, doctor. I think that would help... please go ahead.

How you give bad news really matters to the patient. Attending a course on this and sitting in with bereavement and cancer counsellors are important ways to acquire the necessary skills.

Top tip: Do's and don'ts of breaking bad news

Do	Don't
• Have the facts to hand	• Give too much information at one time
• Check if the patient wants anyone else present	• Give inappropriate reassurance
• Clarify what the patient knows or suspects	• Answer questions unless you have the facts to hand
• Be prepared to follow the patient's agenda	• Hurry the consultation • Use euphemisms
• Observe and acknowledge the patient's emotional reactions	• Stop emotional expressions from the patient
• Check patient's understanding of what you are saying	• Agree to relative's request to withhold information from the patient

THE ANGRY PATIENT OR RELATIVE

Overall, the aim is to resolve conflict positively. In reality, you would pay attention to the environment, e.g. move the patient to a quiet area, as the angry patient with an audience will be less likely to accept your point of view. However, in the OSCE scenario such insight cannot be demonstrated, but the following techniques must be deployed and demonstrated to the examiner.

Top tip: Respect

The use of the person's name in a respectful way (i.e. not forename) in your reply can ease the situation, i.e. Mr Smith, Mrs Jones.

The common causes for anger in a patient include delayed appointments, missed diagnosis, lack of therapeutic success and several forms of miscommunications. The anger may be directed at you, a colleague or an establishment.

An angry patient often triggers the doctor's own fight-or-flight responses and a host of other responses, including annoyance and exasperation. However, an appropriate approach can often defuse the anger and re-establish effective communication with the patient. Many clinicians adopt the approach of disregarding the anger and 'acting normal' or simply attempting to placate the patient without an attempt at understanding the underlying cause of anger – both of these strategies are likely to aggravate the patient, leading to further deterioration of the situation. We show a constructive approach to managing an angry patient.

STEP I: LISTEN: 'GET CURIOUS; NOT FURIOUS'

Let the patient speak her mind without interruption. The fundamental rule is that the patient's story needs to be heard. Your genuine 'curiosity' about what has angered the patient is the first step in resolving the situation. By staying curious, you can avoid being defensive and expressing opinions before the patient finishes her story. You should aim to find out the specifics of the story by encouraging the patient to give the details. You need to remain calm and establish eye contact, get the patient to sit down and try to adopt a similar posture to the patient (mirroring) without an aggressive pose.

Example of good practice in getting a patient to explain why she is angry

Mrs Patel is angry that she spent over an hour trying to park in the hospital car park and now has been told off by the receptionist for being late.

Mrs Patel: Damn it! This place is not here to serve patients! It's crazy that one has pay for the car park and still wait for an hour to find a spot to put your car.

Doctor: Sorry to hear that Mrs Patel…I see you had a tough time trying to find a spot to park. (**echoing**) Having to wait for an hour for a parking spot is a long time. I can see how that would be frustrating. (**empathising**)

Mrs Patel: … and the receptionist was rude. It seems rudeness is an attribute required to work in this place.

Doctor: I am sorry to hear that. Please tell me more about what the receptionist said to you. (maintaining **curiosity**)

(Mrs Patel describes the events.)

STEP 2: EMPATHISE AND DEAL WITH EMOTIONS

Empathy is defined as the identification with and understanding of another's situation, feelings, thoughts and motives. By displaying understanding and concern, you can help the person feel understood. Listening and 'putting yourself in another's shoes' are approaches that lead to empathy. One extremely useful and effective technique is 'echoing', i.e. paraphrasing the patient's comments to convey that you have heard and are seeking to understand. All these approaches are illustrated below.

It is important to encourage expression of feelings – emotions. Concentrate upon dealing with the patient's feelings and avoid rationalising. Acknowledge and validate the emotion so the angry patient feels that you are listening to her, e.g. 'You seem very angry?' Demonstrate your understanding: 'I can see how angry you are about what happened' and 'It must be hard for you'.

> Top tip!
>
> Concentrate upon dealing with the person's feelings and avoid rationalising as this approach is likely to inflame the situation, i.e. an 'explanation' is unlikely to be taken in and may come across as an excuse. It is important to encourage expression of feelings. Attempting to defuse anger, ignoring it or, worse still, countering it with your own anger will be counterproductive. Acknowledging the patient's right to be angry is the best approach as it will begin the healing process and solidify the clinical relationship.

STEP 3: TAKE AN ACTION (IF APPROPRIATE)

If you are at fault, you may offer an apology. Aim to be an advocate for the patient where possible (even if you are at fault!). Point the patient in the direction of resources, e.g. 'Would it help if I put you in touch with the Patient Advisory Liaison Service?' or 'Please tell me if you wish to make a complaint – I can help you with this'. Ironically, a genuine offer of help often results in the patient not pursuing a formal complaint.

The aforementioned three steps apply as long as the patient is angry but not abusive. With a physically abusive patient, you should remove yourself from the scene and call for help. There is no reason for you to tolerate or try to empathise with a verbally abusive patient – the correct approach is to terminate the consultation but with an offer to help: 'Mrs Patel, I really want to listen and understand your concern, but I can't do that if you continue to use inappropriate language'.

DISAGREEMENT BETWEEN PATIENT AND DOCTOR

Disagreements between patients and doctors regarding precise diagnosis and therapy, and occasionally prognosis, are common. Such disagreements can result in non-compliance with tests, medications and appointments, a search for second opinion(s) and non-conventional therapies and, on occasion, even complaints. The abundance of health information (and mis-information) from magazines, the Internet and medical guidelines often results in patients forming ideas about diagnosis and treatment before they step into a doctor's office. How should you deal with these? We illustrate some principles with the example in the box nearby.

> Examples of dealing with disagreement between doctor and patient
>
> Mr and Mrs Khan seek a consultation with you for a 4-year history of infertility. The clinical history (of infrequent periods), androgenic hormone profile and typical ultrasound appearances indicate PCOS. You suggest clomiphene treatment after semen analysis and tubal assessment. However, Mrs Khan pulls a magazine from her handbag and shows you a story about a woman who had healthy twins following treatment with herbal medicine and acupuncture. There are three potential approaches you can take: we recommend the last of these three!

Approach 1

'This is nonsense! Chinese medicine and acupuncture will not correct anovulation. Don't waste your time and money on these please, Mrs Khan'.

Approach 2

'Yes… why not? Let's find a local herbalist for you'.

Approach 3

'Can I make a copy of this article? I would like to look into the merits of this article to see if there is anything in it that can help you. I am glad that you are looking into these issues. However, I must confess that herbal medicine and acupuncture are not recognised treatments for women who do not ovulate. So, the likelihood is that the woman in this magazine article got lucky, and her pregnancy may be unrelated to the treatment she received'.

Outright rejection of a patient's suggestion (as in Approach 1) is likely to set you and your patient on a war path where there will be little common ground. She may seek to go to a doctor who agrees with her ideas about how she should be treated or simply go to the herbalist, rejecting your advice.

Approach 2 is unethical (unless you yourself believe in her approach, in which case there is no disagreement) as you should maintain your professional integrity and role as the patient's advocate, acting in her best interest. Approach 3 offers the middle way.

However, what if she still disagrees with you? Read on.

Mrs Khan: I hear you doctor, but I have so many friends who have now benefited from herbal medicine and acupuncture.

Doctor: I understand, Mrs Khan. Could I please find out more about what you know about these therapies, and how you feel they may help you. Your thoughts may help me in helping you. (**eliciting ICE – ideas, concerns and expectations**)

Mrs Khan: Thank you, doctor. I think the herbs and acupuncture will readjust my hormone levels; that is bound to help my ovaries to release eggs, don't you agree? In fact, I have seen an herbalist already, who has recommended a course of treatment. I hope to start this treatment next week, but I wanted to chat to you before that.

Doctor: OK, Mrs Khan, I see that you have really looked into this approach, and have a lot of faith in it. From scientific data, I have the view that the best treatment for you is clomiphene. I am anxious for you to start clomiphene sooner rather than later, as your advancing age is an important factor in reducing your fertility prospects. So, let me suggest a middle way: You try herbal medicine for 3 months, and if there is no joy, we will start clomiphene?

Mrs Khan: Great! I am very happy with that plan doctor.

When a patient has firm views, you can gently challenge these and try to negotiate a course of action. However, there is no point in trying or coerce the patient into accepting something she does not wish. A patient has the right to autonomy and self-determination. However, if the patient chooses a path that is harmful to her, then you should communicate the facts firmly but empathetically. In the end, you may 'agree to disagree' and such consultations should be carefully documented. Recommending a second opinion in such situations is considered good practice.

When a patient's suggestions are unlikely to harm her, then it is reasonable to make concessions and find a middle way (as in the earlier example).

DISCLOSING MEDICAL ERRORS AND COMPLICATIONS

Research shows that medical errors, complications and 'near misses' are common. Medical defence lawyers have encouraged generations of clinicians not to get involved in disclosing medical errors and certainly not offering apologies for fear of litigation. However, the General Medical Council is clear on this issue: the recommendation is that after an adverse event, a full and honest explanation and an apology, if appropriate, should be provided routinely. There are several good reasons for this. There is now good evidence that disclosure of medical errors can in fact reduce the overall rates of litigation! However, the more important reason is that it helps the patient to handle and to come to terms with the complication. How do you achieve this difficult task? As often cliched, sorry is often the hardest word to say. We take you through this step by step.

STEP 1: PREPARE YOURSELF

Many organisations have a 'disclosure policy', and you should familiarise yourself with this and aim to work within the framework provided by such policies. For example, it may be necessary to involve a risk or clinical governance manager before disclosure about serious events that took place. Find out as much as you can about the complications and their implications, as well as the specific circumstances of the error. Find out what steps need to be taken if the patient is still at risk from the error or complication.

STEP 2: PREPARE THE PATIENT

Start with warning notes, e.g.:

- 'I am afraid I have some upsetting news for you'. **(warning note 1)**
- 'There was a complication at the time of the surgery'. **(warning note 2)**
- 'We caused an injury to the ureter, the tube that connects your kidney to the bladder, during the surgery'. **(communication of the error)**

STEP 3: COMMUNICATE THE ERROR

This needs to be done with honesty and be limited to the information truly known at that point in time. As unpleasant as it may be for the doctor and patient, uncertainties will need to be shared. Unnecessary speculation should be avoided.

STEP 4: APOLOGISE, IF THAT IS THE CORRECT RESPONSE

It is perfectly acceptable to say 'I am sorry'. This statement does not necessarily reflect an admission of liability – it can also be an empathetic response to the patient's predicament.

Disclosure can of course result in litigation whether 'I am sorry' is said or not. Furthermore, non-disclosure itself is now considered a primary reason for litigation. Thus, a full disclosure, with an apology if necessary, is the proper approach to take as it is likely to achieve the primary objective of helping the patient deal with the complication and its consequences.

STEP 5: GIVE EVIDENCE THAT YOU ARE TAKING STEPS

Studies show that patients who have suffered complications seek reassurance that steps will be taken to minimise the occurrence of such complications. Often, it is sufficient to explain that the matter will be investigated and appropriate changes made. Offer to keep the patient informed.

To err is human. Errors and complications will always remain part of clinical medicine, no matter how hard we try to avoid them. An honest approach is the best way when such events occur.

Summary of approach to specific communication and counselling stations

Giving bad news
- Prepare.
- Give a warning note (or two).
- Play it straight.
- Be responsive and repeat as often as necessary.
- Give (appropriate) hope.

Angry patient
- 'Get curious, not furious'.
- Empathise and deal with emotions.
- Take action (if appropriate).

Disagreement between patient and doctor
- Challenge (gently but firmly).
- Negotiate but avoid coercion.
- Compromise if appropriate.
- Consideration of seeking a second opinion in such situations is good practice.

BETTER WORDS AND PHRASES FOR LAY COMMUNICATION

It is remarkably easy not to say what you mean.

(Appleton, BMJ 1994)

Research shows that patients are often confused by their doctor's language (Figure 3.1). For example, a study found that only 60% of cancer patients understood that the term 'metastasis' meant cancer was spreading and only around half knew the term 'remission' meant there was no detectable sign of cancer. One way to improve your chances of helping a patient understand what you are telling her is to choose your words and phrases carefully. How would you explain to a woman the terms 'choroid plexus cysts' or 'trophoblastic disease'? 'Jargon Buster' over the next few pages will benefit your patients and improve your chances in the OSCE.

If you think of a word or phrase that you find particularly troublesome to explain to your patient, we suggest you track down a patient information leaflet on the subject of that word or phrase and in it you are likely to find a way of expressing the word or phrase in plain English (Table 3.1).

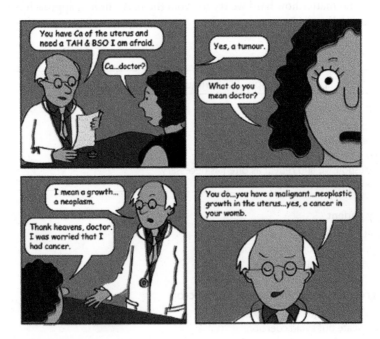

Figure 3.1 Medical jargon.

Table 3.1 Jargon buster

Jargon	Lay explanation
Abruption	A (often sudden) breaking-off of the afterbirth from the womb
Adenomyosis	Womb thickening due to tissues which should only be found in the inner lining of the womb being present in the actual muscle of the womb
AFP (alpha-fetoprotein)	A blood protein that helps to estimate the chance of conditions like Down syndrome
Amniocentesis	A specialised test that involves taking a sample of fluid from the womb with a needle and examining it in the laboratory to see whether the baby has any serious conditions. It is a diagnostic test, which means that it can tell with almost certainty whether or not the baby has got a particular condition
Anembryonic pregnancy	Empty pregnancy sac
Anencepahly	A condition in which the brain and skull of the baby do not form
Anterior colporrhaphy	An operation to correct the bulging of the bladder into the vagina
Antiphospholipid syndrome	A disorder of the immune system in which there can be clotting within arteries or veins, miscarriages and a variety of other problems, some life-threatening
Biophysical profile (BPP) scoring	An ultrasound test to assess the condition of the baby. The BPP measures the baby's heart rate, muscle tone, movement, breathing and the amount of amniotic fluid around the baby
Cerebral palsy	A group of conditions in which the baby's brain is damaged before, during or after birth. Affected children can have various disabilities, including problems with thinking, speech, movement, coordination and learning
Choriocarcinoma	Cancer of the afterbirth (placental) tissues
Choroid plexus cyst	Collection of fluid in cysts in the part of the brain which makes the fluid that cushions the brain and spinal cord. This is a normal ultrasound finding in most women. In some instances, it can indicate a chromosomal (see Chromosomes below) condition in the baby, with an extra copy of chromosome 18
Chorionic villus sampling	A specialised test that involves taking a small piece of afterbirth tissue from the womb with a needle and examining it in the laboratory to see whether the baby has any serious conditions. It is a diagnostic test, which means that it can tell with almost certainty whether or not the baby has got a particular condition
CIN (cervical carcinoma in situ)	A condition in which the neck of the womb (cervix) has cells that are not normal – these cells have a chance of becoming cancer, so the neck of the womb needs to be monitored or treated
Colposcopy	A detailed examination of the neck of the womb with an instrument which provides magnified views

(Continued)

Table 3.1 (*Continued*) Jargon buster

Jargon	Lay explanation
Chromosomes	Thread-like structures in the cells that are the 'building blocks of life', containing the genes; there are 46 of them in humans
Colposuspension	An operation to treat urinary leakage, by providing special support to the bladder and the tube that connects the bladder to the outside (urethra)
CTG	A test that assesses the baby's condition by recording the baby's heart rate. It also records the contractions of the womb
Cytology	Laboratory examination of cells (e.g. from the neck of the womb)
Cystoscopy	An examination of the bladder and the passageway that takes urine from the bladder to the outside (urethra) with a special telescope-like instrument
Cystic fibrosis	An inherited condition in which the body produces thick sticky mucus that damages lungs and other organs
Cystocoele	A condition in which the bladder bulges into or through the vagina
Cystourethrocoele	A condition in which the bladder and the passageway that takes urine from the bladder to the outside bulge through the vagina
Deep venous thrombosis	A blood clot forming in a large vein, like the veins in the leg or thigh. The blood clot can break off and travel in the circulation and can become lodged in the brain, lungs, heart or other area, severely damaging that organ
Diagphramatic hernia	A birth defect in which there is a hole in the diaphragm, the muscle that separates the chest from the tummy (abdomen); this hole allows slipping of the bowel into the chest, causing distress with breathing
Down syndrome	A condition that is most commonly caused by an extra copy of chromosome 21 (see Chromosomes), in which the child has a typical facial appearance, learning difficulties as well as other complications such as heart defect
Dyskaryosis	A smear finding in which there are changes in the appearance of the cells that cover the neck of the womb (cervix). It is not cancer, but in some women, it can become cancer over a period of time; thus, it requires monitoring or treatment
Electrocardiogram (ECG)	A heart trace
Eclampsia A Greek word meaning 'bolt from the blue'	It is a serious complication of pregnancy characterised by convulsions or fits. It is associated with high blood pressure and protein in the urine (pre-eclampsia)
Echocardiogram	An ultrasound test of the heart that gives information about any defects, such as holes in the heart and the pumping action of the heart

(*Continued*)

Table 3.1 (*Continued*) Jargon buster

Jargon	Lay explanation
Edwards syndrome	A condition that is caused by an extra copy of chromosome 18 (see Chromosomes); very few babies survive this condition; when they survive, they can have serious physical and learning disabilities
Epidural	Injection of pain-killing and anaesthetic drugs through a catheter (a tube) placed in the small of the back, going into the space outside the coverings that surround the spinal cord
Embryo	A life at very early stages of development. *Note*: 'embryo' often refers to life from fertilisation to 8 weeks; after 8 weeks, the term 'foetus' is often used
Endometrium	The inner lining of the womb
Endometrial polyp	A 'finger-like projection' or 'fleshy swelling' in the inner lining of the womb
Endometriosis	A condition in which tissues that normally line the womb (endometrium) are found elsewhere, like internal lining of the abdomen (tummy)
Enterocoele	A condition in which the bowels bulge into or through the vagina
Episiotomy	A surgical cut in the vagina and surrounding skin to make room for the vaginal delivery of a baby
Fibroids	A fibroid is a benign (non-cancerous) growth in the womb. It can occur anywhere in the womb and can vary from pea-sized to the size of a melon
Gastroschisis	A condition in which the intestines and sometimes other organs bulge through a hole in the foetal abdomen (tummy)
Group B streptococcus (GBS)	A bacterial infection that can be passed to a baby during delivery. It can cause severe infection in a newborn baby. However, it is not a sexually transmitted infection and outside pregnancy many women have the bacteria without it causing any harm to them
Genes	Genes are 'building blocks of life' which code for human characteristics
Human chorionic gonadotrophin (hCG)	A 'pregnancy hormone' that is produced by the afterbirth tissues (placenta)
Histology	Assessment of tissues in the laboratory with a microscope
HPV screening	Testing for viruses that can cause abnormal cells which, in turn, can lead to cancer in the neck of the womb (if left untreated)
Hystero-contrast-sonography (HyCoSy)	An ultrasound test to check whether the fallopian tubes are blocked or open, by putting a special dye through a catheter (plastic tube) placed in the womb
Hysterosalpingography (HSG)	An X-ray test to check whether the fallopian tubes are blocked or open, by putting a special dye through a catheter (plastic tube) placed in the womb

(Continued)

Table 3.1 (*Continued*) Jargon buster

Jargon	Lay explanation
Hysterosocopy	A test to look inside the womb using a narrow tube-like telescope
Hydrosalpinx	A blocked, dilated, fluid-filled fallopian tube, usually caused by a previous tubal infection
Hydrophic foetus	An abnormal accumulation of fluid in the baby, e.g., in the lungs, around the heart and in the abdomen
ICSI	ICSI is a technique sometimes used in IVF (see IVF below) in which one sperm is injected directly into one egg in order to fertilise it
IVF	An assisted reproductive technique in which the ovaries are stimulated with drugs to produce a large number of eggs which are collected from the ovaries with a needle, to be inseminated with the partner's sperm in a test tube to create embryos which are then transferred into the woman's womb to give the couple a chance of pregnancy
Karyotype	The complete set of chromosomes (see Chromosomes) inside the nucleus of a cell
Laparoscopy	A keyhole operation to look inside the abdomen and pelvis using a narrow tube-like telescope
Laparotomy	A surgical incision on the abdomen to look and treat inside the abdomen or pelvis
Lichen sclerosis	A condition in which the skin around the vagina (vulva) becomes thin, white, shiny and often itchy; the condition is important as it has a small chance of giving rise to cancer
LLETZ (large loop excision of the transformation zone); loop cone biopsy	An operation to remove a small piece of the neck of the womb with the aim of removing abnormal cells from the neck of the womb
Meconium	The green amniotic fluid resulting from the baby opening its bowel while inside the mother's womb
Metastasis	Transfer of cancer from one organ to another
Neural tube defects	Serious birth defects in which the brain, spinal cord or their coverings do not develop completely
Nuchal translucency	A collection of fluid under the skin at the back of a baby's neck, measured with an ultrasound scan at 10–14 weeks' gestation. It is a screening test for Down syndrome
Obstetric cholestasis (cholestasis of pregnancy or intrahepatic cholestasis of pregnancy)	A condition of the mother's liver that is thought to be due to the liver over-responding to pregnancy hormones. It causes itchiness and carries risks to the mother and baby
Ovum	Egg (from the ovary)
Placenta praevia	A pregnancy complication in which the afterbirth (placenta) has attached to the wall of the womb close to or covering the neck of the womb (cervix)
Polyp	(See Endometrial polyp)

(Continued)

Table 3.1 (*Continued*) Jargon buster

Jargon	Lay explanation
Polypectomy	Removal of a polyp (see Endometrial polyp)
Pre-eclampsia	Pre-eclampsia is a serious condition of pregnancy. It is associated with high blood pressure and protein in the urine and can cause complications such as convulsions and damage to organs such as the liver, kidneys and lungs
Proteinuria	Passing protein in the urine
Pulmonary embolism	Simplest explanation: A serious condition in which there are blood clots in the lungs Detailed explanation: A serious condition in which there is a blockage in the blood vessels in the lungs with blood clots; these blood clots often come from dislodged blood clots from other blood vessels such as the veins in the legs
Rectocoele	A condition in which the rectum bulges into or through the vagina
Remission	A state of absence of disease
Respiratory distress syndrome (neonatal)	A breathing disorder in a newborn baby that can sometimes cause serious distress and harm to the baby
Salpingectomy	Removal of fallopian tube(s), often through key-hole surgery
Septicaemia	Blood poisoning with bacterial infection
Smear test	A simple test to collect cells from the neck of the womb (cervix); these cells are tested in the laboratory to see if they have a risk of becoming cancerous
Shoulder dystocia	A serious condition in which the baby's shoulder gets stuck behind the mother's pelvic bone, soon after delivery of the baby's head
Spinal anaesthesia	Injection of pain-killing and anaesthetic drugs through a catheter (a tube) placed in the small of the back, going into the space outside the spinal cord
Spina bifida	(see Neural tube defect). This is the most common neural tube defect, in which the spine does not close properly during early pregnancy development
Stillbirth	Death of a baby inside the womb
Thrombophilia	A range of conditions that results in an individual having 'sticky blood' and thus an increased risk of clots forming in blood vessels, as well as other complications such as miscarriages
Trophoblastic disease, molar pregnancy, hydatidiform mole	Abnormal overgrowth of the afterbirth (see also Choriocarcinoma)
TVT (tension-free vaginal tape)	A TVT operation is performed to help women with incontinence. Two small cuts are made on the lower part of the tummy and another small cut in the vagina. A special tape is then passed through these cuts to form a sling around the tube that lets urine flow out of the bladder (urethra)

(Continued)

Table 3.1 (*Continued*) Jargon buster

Jargon	Lay explanation
Umbilical Doppler test	An ultrasound test of blood flow through the umbilical cord of the baby. The test gives information on the baby's well-being, which often helps us decide on the timing of delivery of the baby
Urodynamic testing	A test performed for a detailed understanding of the way the bladder functions by evaluating urine flow, pressure and volume. A small catheter (tube) will be passed into the bladder via the urethra (the pipe that empties urine from the bladder to the outside) to help us perform this test
Uterine artery Doppler test	An ultrasound test of blood flow through the main blood vessels of the womb. The test gives information on the risks of a pregnant woman developing blood pressure complications (pre-eclampsia) or having a poorly nourished (growth restricted) baby

EXAMPLE QUESTION

Candidate's instructions

This station is a role-play station and will assess your abilities to communicate the foetal diagnosis. You will be assessed using the following domains:

- Patient safety
- Communication with patients and their relatives
- Information gathering
- Applied clinical knowledge

You have been asked to see Mrs Simms, who had a high-resolution ultrasound scan following a very high level of alpha-fetoprotein (AFP) at serum screening. The experienced ultrasonographer who scanned her has told you that she found a large cystic paracranial mass, consistent with an encephalocoele. Mrs Simms is not aware of the diagnosis yet. You are expected to break the news to Mrs Simms and to counsel her. You will have an examiner observing your consultation.

Simulated role-player's instructions

You are Mrs Simms. You have just had an ultrasound scan following a very high level of AFP at serum screening. The ultrasonographer who scanned you has told you nothing but has sent you to see the obstetrician to discuss the scan result.

The candidate (obstetrician) is required to explain the scan result to you and to break the bad news.

Questions you should ask during the consultation:

1. Is this due to my smoking? I knew I should have given up.
2. Are you sure about this diagnosis?

3. With a cyst outside the brain, would vaginal delivery still be possible?
4. Is this genetic? Will I get this again?

Marking

Patient Safety

- Checks the patient's awareness and knowledge of the situation at the beginning of the consultation.
- Offers TOP and explains the process demonstrating knowledge of patient safety.
- Understands the safest mode of delivery – vaginal delivery.

Communication with patients and their relatives

- Demonstrates good communication skills whilst breaking bad news.
- Acknowledges the patient's shock and concern.
- Avoidance of medical jargon throughout, explaining encephalocoele in a simple understandable manner.
- Ensures the patient understands the information communicated and is content with the subsequent management.

Information gathering

- Makes efforts to ascertain what the patient already knows after the ultrasound.
- Attempts to ascertain what the patient understands of the clinical condition.
- Assesses the wish of the patient with regard to termination of pregnancy.

Applied clinical knowledge

- Demonstrates sound knowledge of encephalocoele.
- Demonstrates understanding of additional risks involved with induction of labour in women attempting VBAC.
- Aware of the issues surrounding mode of delivery with encephalocoele.

Examiner's instructions

In this role-play station, the candidate should be able to explain the diagnosis in a clear manner. The candidate should demonstrate that they have the ability appropriately to counsel the patient and discuss management options and to communicate and break bad news. Lastly, the candidate should be able to answer the patient's queries with sympathy and tact.

BASIC COMMUNICATION SKILLS

- Introduction/eye contact/body language.
- Avoidance of medical jargon.
- Information in small doses; repetition of important information; periodical check for understanding.

- Non-directive and sympathetic counselling.
- Allow patient to talk, express concern/shock and ask questions.

DIAGNOSIS AND MANAGEMENT

- Give a warning shot: 'I am afraid the ultrasound has shown a serious finding'.
- Communicate finding without delay: 'The ultrasound shows brain tissues have escaped through a hole in the skull to form a cyst'.
- Discuss the prognosis: 'Difficult to predict the outcome – in terms of survival as well as development. Likely to survive, but with disability' (isolated meningocele – good prognosis; microcephaly associated with brain herniation – very poor prognosis).
- Offer TOP (timing of TOP unlimited by the Abortion Act 1991, Clause E):
  If accepted, discuss details of TOP (intracardiac K; medical TOP – mefipristone and misoprostol); may need surgical evacuation of RPOC; pain relief.
  If TOP declined: routine antenatal care; expect vaginal delivery (but be aware of risk of caesarean section); appointment with paediatric neurologist.

ROLE-PLAYER QUESTION

1. 'Is this due to my smoking? I knew I should have given up'. – No; not related to anything you have or have not done.
2. 'Are you sure about this diagnosis?' – Yes; however, I would be very happy to arrange a second opinion.
3. 'With a cyst outside the brain, would vaginal delivery still be possible?' – In most cases, vaginal delivery is possible – slightly increased risk of caesarean.
4. 'Is this genetic? Will I get this again?' – It may be associated with a genetic problem in this foetus, but that does not mean you or your partner have a genetic condition which would result in recurrent neural tube defects. However, there is an increased risk of NTDs in the future (1/30); thus, high dose folate and high resolution USS in future pregnancies.

SUPPORT, FOLLOW UP AND CLOSING UP

- Summarise.
- Action plan and timelines.
- Information about access to services (including support groups).
- Counselling.
- Offer of further appointments and second opinion.
- Written literature.

CHAPTER 4
RESULTS INTERPRETATION AND MANAGEMENT

You may arrive at a station and be presented with a test result or series of test results to analyse and interpret. Such stations not only examine your ability to extract information from diagnostic test results but also allow an exploration of your knowledge of when and how you would use such tests – the indications, appropriateness and limitations of testing – and how test results will influence your clinical management. Example topics to revise and familiarise yourself with are listed in the box below.

Examples of data interpretation topics

Radiological images (indications, anatomy, pathology, further testing, management)
• Ultrasound (identify transabdominal vs transvaginal)
• Hysterosalpinogram
• MRI/CT scanning

Endoscopic images (indications, anatomy, landmarks, pathology, further testing, management, complications)
• Hysteroscopy
• Cystoscopy
• Laparoscopy

General clinical images (identification and management)
• Pathology
• Complications

Pathology specimens/slides/results
• Lower genital tract microscopy (sexually transmitted infections, bacterial vaginosis, candida)
• Vulval disease
• Cervical cytology
• Cervical intraepithelial neoplasia
• Endometrium (functional, inactive, hyperplastic, cancerous)
• Ovarian cysts

Endocrinology/biochemical results
• β-hCG, FSH, LH, prolactin, oestradiol, day 21 progesterone, androgens – ovarian and adrenal (infertility, polycystic ovaries, pregnancy)
• Ovarian tumour markers
• Seminal fluid analysis
• Other – Thyroid function, diabetes (GTT, random, HbA1C)

Urological
- Urinalysis (urinary tract infection, renal disease, pre-eclamspia – 24-hour protein collection, albumin:creatinine ratio, creatinine clearance)
- Urodynamics

Antenatal tests
- Serological screening tests (including haemoglobinopathies, isoimmunisation, trisomy and infections)
- Ultrasound, including booking, nuchal screening, anomaly, foetal growth scanning, uterine and umbilical Doppler studies, biophysical profiles
- Immunology results – Renal disease/connective tissue disorders and pregnancy
- Pre-eclampsia screen and blood pressure monitoring

Acute obstetrics
- Partogram
- Cardiotocograph
- Foetal blood sample

Acute gynaecology
- Serial β-hCG
- Ultrasound and surgical images (e.g. ectopic, ovarian torsion, trophoblastic disease)

APPROACH TO RESULT INTERPRETATION

1. Greet the examiner and be attentive.
2. Listen to and/or read instructions carefully.
3. Maintain a good posture when reading the test result (put your chair in a position that is comfortable for you and sit forward on the front half of the chair with your feet flat on the floor).
4. Handle any source material presented to you by the examiner sparingly and do not move it/fidget excessively (i.e. do not give the impression that this is the first time you have ever seen such a test/image!).
5. Do not answer immediately even if you are certain of the answer. Pause for a few seconds to allow you to compose your thoughts and formulate an answer. This will convey an impression of a sensible and measured clinician.
6. Engage the examiner and ensure eye contact when responding (there is a tendency to stare at the test result and to ignore the examiner).
7. State what the test/image is, then extract the information/describe the key features in a systematic way (avoid criticising the quality of the image/data provided), identify normal/abnormal results or findings and then give the diagnosis/likely diagnosis supported by your preceding description (e.g. the presence of visible endometriotic peritoneal deposits favours endometriosis as the cause of the filmy tubo-ovarian adhesions, although pelvic inflammatory disease is another possibility). If you do not know the diagnosis, then you will still gain some marks for your description.

Answer the question concisely, but you can expand your answer succinctly if this provides relevant further information demonstrating your understanding (e.g. use of additional, confirmatory tests; suggest what you would normally do when presented with these findings).

If challenged by the examiner, then reconsider your answer, but if you still believe that your initial interpretation or management plan was a good one, then justify your case with supporting statements in a firm but courteous manner. If it is clear you have 'messed up', then acknowledge this gracefully and move on to ensure you concentrate fully on the next case/question.

8. The examiner will then ask further questions based upon the test result or provide further tests to be interpreted.
9. Do not worry if the examiner gives you no feedback when moving between cases as, whilst this is unnerving, they will have been instructed not to provide positive or negative reinforcement.
10. Thank the examiner when leaving the station.

Sample data interpretation station – Urodynamics

Candidate's instructions

At this station, you will have 10 minutes to answer structured questions. You will be presented with several investigation results. You will be asked to interpret these and answer any supplementary questions that the examiner asks which will assess the following domains:

- Communication with colleagues
- Applied clinical knowledge
- Patient safety

Marking

Communication with colleagues

- Explains concepts clearly.
- Evidence of structuring of answers.

Applied clinical knowledge

- Understands the indications of urodynamic studies.
- Understands how to interpret urodynamic studies.
- Understands the treatment of detrusor overactivity and the risks of anticholinergic medications.

Patient safety

- Knows when urodynamic studies are not required.
- Aware of the risks of anticholinergic medications in the presence of voiding difficulties.

Examiner's instructions

This is a structured viva assessing the candidate's ability to interpret the data provided. It also assesses their knowledge regarding the assessment of urinary incontinence by using urodynamics. You should ask the candidate the questions provided in sequence. If required, you can prompt the candidate; however, this should be reflected in your overall assessment.

Structured VIVA questions

Provide the candidate with Result A (Figure 4.1)
   Ask the following questions:

A1. What do lines A, B and C indicate?

A2. What are the indications for performing the above test?

A3. What can cause wandering baselines when there is no real change in the bladder or intra-abdominal pressure?

A4. What is the urodynamic diagnosis in the cystometrogram?

A5. What are the mainstay therapies for the condition?

A6. What are the newer modalities for treating this condition that you are aware of?

A7. What is the significance of a detrusor pressure rise of above 50 cm H$_2$O water?

Provide the candidate with Result B (Figure 4.2)

B1. If the patient also leaked with cough in the above cystometrogram, what would your diagnosis be?

B2. What is the significance of voiding studies in this condition?

Result C (Figure 4.3)

C1. What is the above investigation and what abnormalities can you see?

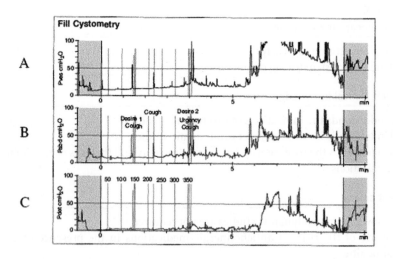

Figure 4.1 Result A.

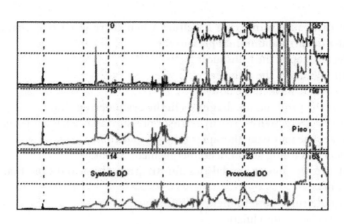

Figure 4.2 Result B.

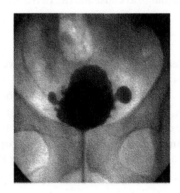

Figure 4.3 Result C.

Answers

Result A

A1. What do lines A, B and C indicate?
- A – Bladder pressure
- B – Rectal pressure which denotes intra-abdominal pressure
- C – Detrusor pressure

A2. What are the indications for performing the above test?
Multichannel filling and voiding cystometry is recommended in women before surgery for urinary incontinence in the following circumstances:
- Clinical suspicion of detrusor overactivity.
- Previous surgery for stress incontinence or anterior compartment prolapse.
- Symptoms suggestive of voiding dysfunction.
- There is a need to demonstrate the presence of specific abnormalities before undertaking complex reconstructive urological procedures.
- Clinical diagnosis is unclear prior to surgery.
- Initial treatment has failed.

A3. What can cause wandering baselines when there is no real change in the bladder or intra-abdominal pressure?
- Rectal drop of the transducer
- Air bubbles in the catheter
- Peristaltic wave in the bowel

A4. What is the urodynamic diagnosis in the cystometrogram?
Detrusor overactivity – rise in detrusor pressure associated with urgency.

A5. What are the mainstay therapies for the condition?
Bladder retraining and anticholinergic medications.

A6. What are the newer modalities for treating this condition that you are aware of?
- Intradetrusor botulinum toxin injection
- Sacral neuronmodulation

A7. What is the significance of a detrusor pressure rise of above 50 cm H_2O water?
Need to rule out neurological cause for the detrusor overactivity, e.g. multiple sclerosis.

Result B

B1. If the patient also leaked with cough in the above cystometrogram, what would your diagnosis be?
Provoked detrusor overactivity as the leak would be associated with detrusor pressure rise. Remember that for urodynamic stress incontinence, the incontinence has to be demonstrable without the detrusor pressure rise.

B2. What is the significance of voiding studies in this condition?
To rule out pre-existing voiding difficulties and as baseline prior to starting anticholinergics, etc., as they can be associated with urinary retention.

Result C

C1. What is the above investigation and what abnormalities can you see?
- Videocystourethrogram taken at videourodynamics.
- Abnormalities seen: trabeculation, diverticuli and vesicoureteric reflux on the right side.

CHAPTER 5
CRITICAL APPRAISAL OF THE MEDICAL LITERATURE AND AUDIT

Critical appraisal of medical literature is a core competency in various modules within the RCOG curriculum. Critical appraisal questions are likely to fit into one of the five categories:

1. Therapy studies (randomised controlled studies)
2. Diagnostic studies (test accuracy studies)
3. Systematic reviews and meta-analyses
4. Patient information leaflets
5. Audits

It is possible to be presented with other types of studies, e.g. ones on prognosis (cohort study), aetiology (case-control or cohort studies) or efficiency (economic evaluations) but is unlikely.

Previously, during preparatory stations, MRCOG candidates would be asked to appraise medical literature or design an audit to then present findings or suggestions at the subsequent station. There are no longer any preparatory stations in the current format of the MRCOG Part 3 examination. However, it is still feasible that you could be asked to interpret a short abstract, appraise a short patient information leaflet or be asked to describe how you would design an audit. Therefore, if the need arises, the principles provided in this chapter can be modified to address all these different types of tasks.

WHY APPRAISE THE MEDICAL LITERATURE?

Many papers published in medical journals have serious methodological flaws and most are irrelevant for everyday clinical practice. Although many of you are in the 'user' mode when you look for evidence to support practice, you cannot always find up-to-date and valid pre-appraised summaries and synopses, and it becomes necessary to switch to 'appraiser' mode, roll up your sleeves and try to make sense of the evidence yourself. This process starts with defining the exact clinical question you want answered and finding the relevant paper(s), and only then does appraising them become an issue. However, as you will be given the paper for appraisal in the OSCE, the steps of defining the question, and searching and finding the literature will not be relevant in the exam and are not covered in this chapter.

So, what does appraisal involve? It involves checking the articles for

- Validity (methodological soundness)
- Importance (e.g. is a *statistically* significant reduction in BP of 2 mmHg *clinically* significant?)
- Applicability to your patients

Various checklists exist to help in the appraisal of different types of clinical questions (see www.cebm.net). We cover the important ones in this chapter.

ANATOMY OF A SCIENTIFIC PAPER

Most scientific articles have the IMRAD structure – Introduction (or background), Methods (or materials and methods), Results (or findings) and Discussion. They often have an abstract which is also usually structured as IMRAD. All of these sections are important, but some are more important than others. Which are these? This may seem an academic question, but it is not! If you are struggling to make sense of a lengthy article due to time limitation in your OSCE, you will need to prioritise what you read. We recommend that you prioritise the abstract, methods and results. The *abstract* should give you a quick overview of the paper; the *methods* should tell you what was done in the study, from which you can assess its validity and the *results* should tell you what was found. What about the introduction and the discussion that we know many of you are fond of devoting a lot of time to? If time permits, by all means do read these, but these are secondary to the abstract, methods and results.

GENERAL PRINCIPLES IN APPRAISING A SCIENTIFIC PAPER

Step 1: Introduce

Introduce the paper and your purpose: *I would like to present the appraisal findings of this article by (mention first author) and colleagues, published in (journal name) in (year of publication) on the subject of (subject matter of the paper). I will summarise the appraisal findings, highlighting the study's strengths and weaknesses and conclude with my interpretation of the findings in terms of implications for clinical practice and for research.*

Step 2: Define the exact clinical question asked by the paper

The way to define a clinical question is by using the PICOD structure (Table 5.1). You can often get all elements of PICOD from the abstract, although sometimes it is necessary to go through the Methods section to find all the relevant information.

Table 5.1 PICOD structure to define a clinical question

Component	Example 1	Example 2
P: Population, patient or problem	In women at risk of pre-eclampsia	In pregnant women with swollen legs
I: Intervention (test, treatment or process of care)	Would treatment with low-dose aspirin	Would a Doppler ultrasound be accurate
C: Comparison (placebo, another treatment or the gold standard in a diagnostic accuracy study)	Compared to placebo	Compared to venography as the gold standard
O: Outcome(s)	Lead to reduction in the risk of pre-eclampsia and perinatal mortality?	In diagnosing DVTs?
D: Design of the study	An RCT	A test accuracy study

Once you have identified your PICOD elements, put these together succinctly in a statement for your examiner. For example: *This randomised controlled trial evaluates the effectiveness of low-dose aspirin compared to a placebo on the outcomes of pre-eclampsia and perinatal mortality in women at risk of pre-eclampsia.*

Step 3: Provide details

Now dive deep into the Methods section, particularly looking at the *inclusion and exclusion criteria*. The purpose is to provide more details on PICOD. For example: *In this study high risk women (population) were defined as women with a previous history of pre-eclampsia, chronic hypertension or diabetes and those who had positive uterine artery Doppler at 12–14 weeks gestation. The intervention was aspirin at a dose of 75 mg, started at 14 weeks' gestation and continued until 36 weeks. The primary outcomes were pre-eclampsia, defined as... and perinatal death, defined as... The secondary outcomes were ....*

Step 4: Appraise the study for validity

All the information you need for this will be found in the Methods section. Checklists that will help you with the appraisal of the three common types of articles are provided in the next few pages. It is important to approach your paper with a checklist like these in your mind. Then, your reading of the article will be purposeful and focused as you gather the facts to answer the questions in the checklist. You can then summarise the output from this exercise. For example: *This is a randomised, allocation-concealed, placebo-controlled, double-blind study. Randomisation was achieved with the use of a computer-generated random number list; allocation concealment was accomplished by placing the treatment allocation in opaque envelopes; both the clinician providing the care and the patient were blinded, making the study double-blind. The analysis was by intention-to-treat and the follow-up rate was excellent, with data being available on over 95% of those who were randomised. Thus, the methods of this trial are excellent.*

Of course, if there are any weaknesses in the methods, you will highlight these also. This step is the backbone of your appraisal. Do a good job with it and do not rush it!

Step 5: Provide the findings

You will find all that you need to address this step in the Results section and the tables and figures of the article. Table 1 in most articles is where researchers summarise data on demographic and baseline characteristics of the populations being compared – start with this. Then move on to providing the study findings. Provide confidence intervals around the findings where these are provided. For example: *The baseline characteristics between the aspirin and placebo group were similar. The main findings were that there was a reduction in pre-eclampsia risk, with a relative risk (RR) of 0.6 and a 95% confidence interval (CI) from 0.5 to 0.8. The study also found that….*

Step 6: Put the study findings in the context of the existing evidence

A judgement can almost never be made about the value of an intervention or test based on one paper alone – you need to weigh up the balance of evidence. For this step, you may find the Discussion section of the article helpful, if the authors have taken the trouble to place their study in the context of existing evidence. Unfortunately, the Discussion section of articles is generally abused by authors: they shamelessly fill it with irrelevant curiosities that they were unable to place elsewhere and often put spin on their findings. So, skim through the Discussion, but if you find that the authors have written about previous studies on this subject, stop and take this in. Hopefully, using the information in the Discussion and your pre-existing knowledge, you can put the study in context. If you cannot, you may have to state to the examiner that you would want to find out more about what other studies on this subject show before you could decide on whether the evidence should be incorporated into clinical practice. Your efforts should produce something of this sort: *The findings from the study are consistent with over 40 other studies summarised in a Cochrane review.*

Step 7: Make your recommendation for practice and research

There is no point in appraising a paper unless you come to some judgement about whether it is appropriate for guiding clinical practice or further research. Steps 4, 5 and 6 will contribute to your judgement: *As this is a high quality study that shows substantial reduction in pre-eclampsia and perinatal death, and the findings are consistent with other studies on this subject, I will recommend aspirin therapy to women at risk of pre-eclampsia* [clinical implication]. *Further research may be required to examine the role of aspirin in other high risk groups such as those with renal disease* [research implication].

APPRAISING A THERAPY PAPER (RANDOMISED CONTROLLED TRAILS)

Checklist to appraise a therapy article

I. Are the results valid?
- Is the assignment of patients randomised? (*appropriate methods are: random number tables and computer-generated random numbers*)
- Is the allocation of patient concealed? (*appropriate methods are opaque envelopes, third-party randomisation, distant [telephone or the Internet] allocation*)
- Are patients, health workers and study personnel 'blind' to treatment?
- Are patients analysed in the groups to which they were randomised? (*'Intention-to-treat' analysis*)
- Are all patients who entered the trial properly accounted for and attributed at its conclusion?
- Is follow-up complete?
- Are the groups similar at the start of the trial? (normally presented in Table I of the article)
- Aside from the experimental intervention, are the groups treated equally?
- Was the study adequately powered?*
- Was ethical approval obtained for the study?*

2. What are the results (i.e. their importance)?
- How large is the treatment effect? (*reported as relative risks, odds ratios, absolute risks or numbers needed to treat [NNT]*)
- How precise is the treatment effect? (*95% confidence interval*)

3. Will the results help me in caring for my patients (applicability)?
- Can the results be applied to my patients?
- Are all clinically important outcomes considered?
- What are the likely benefits? Are they worth the potential harms and costs?

*These items do not strictly relate to 'validity'; nevertheless, they are important and should be part of the appraisal process.

APPRAISING A DIAGNOSIS ARTICLE

Checklist to appraise a diagnosis article

1. Are the results valid?
- Does the patient sample include an appropriate spectrum of patients to whom the test will be applied in clinical practice?
- Were the test and reference (gold) standard results obtained by assessors blinded to each other?
- Did everyone get *both* the test and the reference standard?
- Is the test described fully?
- Is the reference standard described fully?

2. What are the results?
- What are the results? (*sensitivity, specificity, predictive values or likelihood ratios*)
- What is their precision? (*95% confidence intervals*)

3. Will the results help me in caring for my patients?
- Are the results applicable to my patients?
- Will the results change my management?
- Will patients be better off as a result of the test?

APPRAISING A SYSTEMATIC REVIEW OR META-ANALYSIS

Checklist to appraise a systematic review or meta-analysis

1. Are the results valid?
- Does the article address a clearly focused question? (*i.e. are the PICOD elements clearly defined?*)
- Are the criteria used to select articles for inclusion appropriate?
- Is the literature search comprehensive? (MEDLINE, EMBASE, Cochrane Library, CINRHL, searches for abstracts, hand-searching, etc.)
- Is the validity of the included studies appraised? (*using checklists like those given above*)
- Did two or more reviewers extract the data independently?
- Are the results consistent from study to study?
- Is there an assessment for publication bias? (*e.g. funnel plot analysis*)

2. What are the results?
- What are the results of the study?
- How precise are the results? (*95% confidence intervals*)

3. Will the results help me in caring for my patients?
- Can the results be applied to my patient care?
- Are all clinically relevant outcomes considered?
- Are the benefits worth the harms and costs?

APPRAISING A PATIENT INFORMATION LEAFLET

A patient information leaflet can be appraised under the broad headings of validity, clarity, credibility, currency and format.

At the end of the assessment, do not forget to provide an overall judgement on the quality of the information leaflet. For example, you may state: *In summary, this information leaflet has many strengths* [name a few] *and a few minor weaknesses* [name a few], *and thus with minor modifications, I would be happy to use it with the patients that I look after.*

Checklist to appraise an information leaflet

- Is the aim clearly stated?
- **Validity:**
  Is the information accurate and comprehensive?
  Are the sources of information given? (e.g. patient information leaflet may have been based on a guideline, literature review or a consensus process)
- **Clarity and presentation:**
  Is the language simple and non-medical?
  Are there annotated diagrams?
  Have boxes and bullet points been used?
  Have the authors used a question and answer format?
  Have they provided useful summaries? (ideally, at the beginning and at the end)
  Has there been good use of colour?
- **Credibility:**
  Is authorship of the patient information leaflet given? (it is not good enough to state, 'This patient information leaflet was produced by "x" or "y" society' – the actual authors' names should be provided)
  Is there a 'conflict of interest' declaration stated by any authors? (this is particularly important for any patient information leaflet that carries recommendations for commercial products, including specific drugs)
- **Currency:**
  Is there a creation date?
  Is there an expiry or revision date?
- **Format:** Can the leaflet be folded to fit into a handbag? (*it needs to be A5 size or smaller*)
- Is there a section on 'Further information and help'?

APPRAISING AN AUDIT

If you understand the six steps of an audit, then designing or appraising an audit becomes an easy task. The six steps are detailed below, using an audit of colposcopy referrals from primary care to secondary care as an example where appropriate.

Step 1: Define criteria and standards

Many people are confused by the difference between the terms criterion and standard. The difference is best illustrated with an example. A 'criterion' for a colposcopy referral audit may be: 'women with moderate dyskaryosis should be referred after 1 abnormal smear'. A 'standard' related to that criterion may be: 'At least 90% of women with a moderate dyskaryosis should be seen within 4 weeks of referral'.

Criteria and standards often come from national or professional body guidelines (e.g. the RCOG Green Top Guidelines often provide 'auditable standards'), policy statements, reviews of practice (i.e. previous audits or surveys) or consensus by stakeholders.

Step 2: Measure current practice

- Decide whether this needs to be
  Prospective (time consuming but provides more complete data; however, this approach may suffer from the Hawthorne effect of improvement in practice while the audit is being conducted) or
  Retrospective (quicker to do, but there may be a great deal of missing data).
- Consider the **sampling** frame – all in a defined period, random, or arbitrary?
- Consider the **sample size** (balance between precision and feasibility). (People often discuss 'power calculation'. This is an irrelevant phrase in the context of audits, as audits are not designed to test hypothesis, and consideration of type I and type II errors and power do not apply to audits.)
- **Design (and pilot) the data collection form/pro-forma** (make it as simple as possible – just collecting the essential data for the audit and not looking for 'interesting facts' and burdening the data collectors).
- Decide on **data entry** into a database (e.g. Excel).

Step 3: Analyse data

- Consider possibility of sampling/selection bias.
- Quantitative analysis (e.g. what proportion of women with moderate dyskaryosis were referred to the colposcopy unit?).
- Qualitative analysis (why were some missed?).
- Decide on the format of presentation of data (e.g. pie charts, bar charts, proportions).

Step 4: Present results

- Anticipate reactions.
- Do this sensitively; do not assign personal blame ('hard on issues; soft on individuals').
- Use various methods, e.g.:
  Audit meetings

Hospital e-mails
Letters
'Quality improvement journals' (if your audit has a wider relevance outside your own setting)

Step 5: Identify (as well as disseminate and implement) strategies to improve the care

- Involve all stakeholders.
- Consider revising guidelines.
- Consider multifaceted approaches.
- Consider resource implications.

Step 6: Close the audit loop

Plan a re-audit at an appropriate time to check the changes have been made (process audit) and outcomes are improved (outcome audit).

CHAPTER 6
EQUIPMENT, SURGERY AND PRACTICAL PROCEDURES

This chapter addresses common surgical interventions in O&G relevant to the MRCOG Part 3 examination. When asked to discuss patient management in relation to surgical intervention, you should consider relevant pre-, peri- and post-operative factors. This chapter summarises key issues in terms of pre-operative workup, description and use of surgical equipment, generic operative technique and approach for specific procedures, and also how to prevent and recognise complications.

PRE-OPERATIVE ASSESSMENT AND CONSENT

Pre-operative assessment

Once a surgical intervention has been decided upon, thought must turn to the pre-operative preparation of patients in order to minimise complications. Hospital admission should be kept to a minimum both for the convenience of patients and to reduce risk of hospital-acquired infections (e.g. methicillin-resistant *Staphylococcus aureus* [MRSA]) and venous thromboembolism (VTE). In addition, consider the following:

- General advice where relevant (e.g. stop smoking, reduce weight).
- Prophylaxis against infection.
- VTE score and prophylaxis (see Section "Venous thromboembolism").
- Physical status. A five-category pre-operative classification system from the American Society of Anaesthesiologists (ASA) has been widely adopted:
  - I. Healthy patient
  - II. Mild systemic disease (no functional limitations)
  - III. Severe systemic disease (definite functional limitations)
  - IV. Severe systemic disease that is a constant threat to life
  - V. Moribund patient who is not expected to survive without the operation
- Pre-operative investigation will be dictated by the type of procedure (elective vs emergency; major vs minor operation) and the ASA classification of physical status. Most procedures in O&G require only a full blood count (FBC) and a blood group and save depending upon the risk of bleeding and pre-operative haemoglobin level.

Pre-operative investigations

- *Full blood count* (abnormal uterine bleeding, >60 years old, risk of bleeding during operation, point-of-care testing in operating theatre unavailable)
- *Blood group and save* (significant risk of bleeding/requiring blood transfusion – consider cross-match if risk of bleeding high, pre-operative anaemia or rapid cross-matching unavailable)
- *Coagulation screen* (e.g. taking warfarin, on renal dialysis, liver or vascular disease)
- *Blood gases* (cardiorespiratory disease)
- *Sickle cell test* (ethnicity with higher risk of sickle cell disease or trait)
- *Renal function tests* (>60 years old, diabetes, hypertension, on medications that affect renal function, known renal disease)
- *Pregnancy test* (consider a pregnancy test in all women of reproductive age prior to gynaecological surgery)

Consent

In any discussion pertaining to surgical interventions, the concept of consent cannot be ignored. Candidates must understand the importance legally and ethically of obtaining valid consent prior to medical intervention. The issues around consent have been well documented and are beyond the scope of this revision book. Here we highlight three key principles:

1. If consent is to be considered valid, it must be given voluntarily by an appropriately informed person who has the capacity to consent to the intervention.
2. The clinician providing the treatment or investigation is responsible for ensuring that the patient has given valid consent before treatment.
3. Obtaining consent may be delegated to another suitably trained and qualified health professional as long as they have sufficient knowledge and understanding of the proposed intervention, including the risks involved, so as to provide any information the patient may require.

The RCOG has developed some procedure-specific advice for clinicians, outlining the risks and side effects of common O&G procedures, which should be useful to the prospective MRCOG Part 3 candidate (available at https://www.rcog.org.uk/en/guidelines-research-services/consent/).

The WHO surgical safety checklist should be performed prior to any operation and is currently a 'hot topic'. Any candidate that has spent time in theatre will be expected to be familiar with the components of the checklist. Details of the WHO surgical safety checklist are available at http://www.nrls.npsa.nhs.uk/resources/?entryid45=59860.

FUNDAMENTAL PRINCIPLES OF SURGERY

Patient positioning

Most operative procedures in O&G involve positioning patients to ensure good access to the pelvis and perineum.

- **Trendelenburg position:** supine position with the feet higher than the head (e.g. abdominal hysterectomy).
- **Lithotomy position:** supine position with hips/knees flexed and abducted (e.g. hysteroscopy, vaginal surgery, instrumental delivery).
- **Lloyd-Davies position:** lithotomy position with reduced flexion of the hips (e.g. laparoscopic surgery).

Surgical incisions

Laparotomy in O&G practice uses the following two incisions:

- **Lower transverse** (Pfannensteil = curved; Maylard = curved + rectus muscles cut; Cohen = straight + blunt entry)
- **Vertical** (midline; paramedian)

Compared with a vertical incision, transverse incisions limit exploration of the upper abdomen, are associated with greater blood loss, are more prone to haematoma formation and result in greater paraesthesia of the overlying skin. However, transverse approaches give better cosmetic results, less post-operative pain and are associated with a lower incidence of wound dehiscence and hernia formation.

Be prepared to discuss the rationale, advantages and disadvantages of each type of incision and when you would use them. Remember, you will never be criticised for performing a midline entry, especially where access is likely to be limited (e.g. the obese patient, adhesions are expected – previous surgery, infection, endometriosis).

Rational for abdominal incisions

- Abdominal incisions are based on anatomical principles.
- They must adequately assess to the abdomen.
- They should be capable of being extended if required.
- Ideally, muscles fibres should be split rather than cut.
- Nerves should not be divided.

Suture selection

A suture is any strand of material used to approximate tissue or ligate vessels. The material used should provide uniform tensile strength throughout healing and knot security, induce little tissue reaction (scarring), be resistant to infection, have

Table 6.1 Types of suture commonly used in O&G surgery

Absorbable	Non-absorbable
Surgical gut	Stainless steel (clips)
Polyglactin (Vicryl)	Silk
Polyglycolic acid (Dexon)	Nylon (Dermalon)
Poliglecaprone (Monocryl)	Polypropylene (Prolene)
Polydioxanone (PDS)	Braided synthetics (Dacron)

a favourable absorption profile and be non-allergenic. Sutures are either *absorbable,* providing temporary wound support until the wound heals well enough to withstand normal stress (broken down by enzymatic action or hydrolysis) or *non-absorbable* (Table 6.1).

Sutures are no longer needed when a wound has reached maximum strength. Thus, in general, consider non-absorbable sutures or delayed absorbable sutures for slowly healing tissues (e.g. skin, fascia) and absorbable sutures for rapidly healing tissues (mucous membranes, e.g. peritoneum).

Be prepared to discuss when to use particular types of suture and needle (cutting vs blunt needle point; absorbable vs non-absorbable; monofilament vs multifilament; suture size; patient characteristics, tissues being approximated; when to remove skin sutures).

Electrosurgery

In view of the widespread use of electrosurgery in gynaecological practice, the aspiring MRCOG Part 3 candidate should be able to display an understanding of the fundamental principles and applications of this energy modality. Key points to understand are as follows:

- **Electrical generators.** These convert mains AC electric current (50 Hz) to high-frequency current (200 kHz–3.3 MHz), avoiding muscle contraction and electrocution.
- **Electrical waveforms.** Electrosurgical generators can produce a variety of electrical waveforms. A constant waveform produces a rapid and intense temperature rise (>100°C), which vaporises and easily cuts through tissue (pure cut). If the duty cycle generated is interrupted (an intermittent or modulated waveform), less heat is produced, resulting in different tissue effects (blended cut). As the duty cycle is progressively reduced, cutting (vaporisation) properties wane and desiccation (coagulation providing haemostasis) becomes the dominant tissue effect (80°C–100°C).
- **Heat and tissue effects.** These are produced whenever current flows through tissues and are dependent upon the resistance of the tissues and the density of current flow. Eschar deposited upon electrodes or charring of tissues increases resistance to current flow, whereas the use of a fine electrode, end on, with 'sparking' in close proximity to, rather than direct contact with, tissue and

longer activation times maximises current density and heat production. The 'cutting' waveform can be used to coagulate, and the 'coagulation' waveform can be used to cut, depending upon how the electrode is used.

- **Monopolar vs bipolar circuits.** In bipolar electrosurgery, both the active and return electrode functions occur at the site of surgery, whereas with monopolar diathermy, the current flows through the patient to a more distant return electrode. Bipolar circuits are inherently safer because the current path is confined to the intervening tissue, reducing the risk of stray current and alternate site burns.
- **Safety.** Modern electrosurgical generators have greatly reduced the risks of current diversion and unintended burns. The operator must adopt good practice (e.g. store electrodes in insulated holders, activate electrodes only under direct vision in close or direct proximity to tissues, use the lowest available effective power setting and, ideally, bipolar circuits). Laparoscopic surgery requires a higher level of vigilance to avoid the additional risks of direct coupling (inadvertent contact between the activated electrode and another conducting instrument) and capacitive coupling (use of mixed plastic/metal cannulate preventing dissipation of capacitively coupled electrical energy).

Miscellaneous

Be prepared to discuss other general points relating to surgery, e.g. the need for catheterisation, when to leave drains, types of drain; purpose of post-operative review, duration of stay, discharge and follow-up.

PREVENTING COMPLICATIONS

Anticipate potential problems and arrange adequate time for surgery, help from anaesthetists/urologists/general surgeons, bowel preparation. Common factors associated with an increased risk of surgical complications include the following:

- Risks of surgery vs benefits (remember the Hippocratic Oath)
- Obesity
- Adhesions (previous surgery, infection, endometriosis)
- Pelvic cancer
- Radical surgery

Infection

Surgical site and hospital-acquired infections need to be considered as part of any discussion on operative interventions, an appreciation of the risk of infection and both primary and secondary prevention is important. In O&G practice, the most likely pathogens to be encountered are Gram-negative bacilli, enterococci, Group B streptococci and anaerobes.

Prevention of infection begins pre-operatively by identifying those patient groups at increased risk (diabetics, obese, smokers, steroid use, malnourished, acute admissions) and screening where necessary (see below). Peri-operative measures used to reduce infection risk include the following:

- Use of appropriate antibiotics (up to 1 hour prior to skin incision) to reduce the microbial burden of intraoperative contamination to a level that cannot overwhelm host defences.
- Restricted use of surgical shaves.
- Use of antiseptic agents for pre-operative skin preparation at the incision site (e.g. iodophors, alcohol-containing products and chlorhexidine gluconate).
- Careful surgical technique (minimise tissue trauma).

Information relating to two serious and topical post-operative infections, namely methicillin-resistant MRSA and *Clostridium difficile*, is presented in Sections "Methicillin-resistant *S. aureus*" and "*Clostridium difficile*".

Methicillin-resistant *S. aureus*

Staphylococcus aureus, including MRSA, is found in human skin, particularly in the anterior nares (nose – up to 30% of the population are nasal carriers), axilla (armpit) and perineum (groin). Clinical infection with MRSA occurs either from the patient's own resident MRSA (asymptomatic carrier) or by cross-infection from another person (healthcare worker or visitor [asymptomatic carrier]) or directly/indirectly from a clinically infected patient.

- **Prevention**
  - Screening
  - Hand hygiene (antiseptics, use alcohol-based hand rubs between patients)
  - Regularly clean environment
  - Dress skin wounds
  - Isolate infected patients
- **Screening.** The transmission of MRSA and the risk of MRSA infection can only be addressed effectively if measures are taken to identify MRSA carriers as potential sources and treat them to reduce the risk of transmission. This requires screening of patient populations for MRSA carriage either before or on admission to identify carriers and implement a decolonisation regimen. However, local practice to reduce the risk of MRSA infection (level of screening and decontamination regimens) varies in the absence of consistent, evidence-based advice. Some adopt selective screening of higher risk groups (previously known to be MRSA positive; orthopaedic/cardiothoracic/neurosurgical patients; immunocompromised; admission from nursing homes; emergency admissions) and others employ universal screening.
- **Screening samples.** Anterior nares (nose) – the most common carriage site for MRSA – and most patients positive at other sites have positive results from nose samples (but a small proportion do not). The secondary sites to sample are the axilla and perineum.

- **Decolonisation.** This comprises the use of an antibacterial shampoo and body wash daily (e.g. Aquasept) and the application of an antibacterial nasal cream (e.g. mupirocin nasal ointment) three times a day for 5 days with the aim of eradicating the organism. The purpose of decolonisation is to reduce the risk of both the patient developing an MRSA infection with their own MRSA during medical or surgical treatment and transmission of MRSA to another patient.
- **Treatment of clinical MRSA infection**
  - Isolation (side rooms) to reduce the risk of transmission to other patients
  - Decolonisation regimen
  - Antibiotics, e.g. vancomycin and teicoplanin

Clostridium difficile

This is a spore-forming, Gram-positive bacillus carried in the gastrointestinal tract of a small proportion of adults in the community, with higher rates in hospital patients. Antibiotic-associated colitis caused by *C. difficile* exhibits a spectrum of disease, from diarrhoea through colitis to toxic megacolon and pseudomembranous colitis, which can be fatal.

- **Primary prevention**
  - Restricted use of antibiotics
  - Routine infection control procedures (particularly hand-washing by healthcare staff)
  - Patient education and hand-washing
  - Environmental cleaning, in particular of toilet areas
- **Secondary prevention.** Infection control procedures should be strictly adhered to during an outbreak to prevent cross-infection:
  - Isolation in a room with en suite toilet facilities
  - Hand decontamination for both staff and patients
  - Use of disposable gloves and plastic aprons for the care of patients with diarrhoea
  - Daily cleaning to reduce spore load in the environment, particularly linen and patient equipment
  - Restrict admissions to the unit
- **Management.** Withdrawal of antibiotics and rehydration will resolve most cases. Although antibiotics precipitate the disease, antibiotic therapy with metronidazole and/or vancomycin can be used to resolve it.

Venous thromboembolism

Pelvic surgery is a major risk for VTE. Do not forget to consider prophylaxis against VTE when discussing operative procedures in O&G.

For *gynaecological surgery*, the National Institute for Clinical Excellence (NICE) recommends the following:

- Mechanical prophylaxis using graduated elastic compression stockings and/or intermittent pneumatic compression devices, in the absence of patient-related risk factors.
- Mechanical prophylaxis plus low molecular weight heparin (LMWH) if there are any patient-related risk factors (e.g. age >60 years, obesity [body mass index >30 kg/m^2], personal/family history of VTE, inherited thrombophilias, pregnancy or puerperium, use of oral contraceptives or HRT).
- Do not routinely offer pharmacological or mechanical VTE prophylaxis to patients undergoing a surgical procedure with local anaesthesia by local infiltration with no limitation of mobility.

Other measures to avoid VTE associated with gynaecological surgery

- Early mobilisation.
- Avoid dehydration.
- Advise patients to consider stopping combined oral contraceptives 4 weeks before elective surgery.
- Inform patients that immobility associated with continuous travel of >3 hours in the 4 weeks before or after surgery may increase the risk of VTE.
- Encourage patients to wear stockings from admission until they return to their usual levels of mobility.

Women having a *caesarean section* are at increased risk of VTE. The choice of length of prophylaxis should take into account the risk of VTE (e.g. increased risk with emergency caesarean sections, age >35 years, obesity, medical complications). The Greentop Guideline 37a 'Reducing the risks of venous thromboembolism during pregnancy and the puerperium' should be consulted for details.

MANAGEMENT OF COMMON SURGICAL COMPLICATIONS IN O&G

- **Bladder injury.** Repair in two layers with absorbable sutures + continuous bladder drainage by a suprapubic or transurethral catheter, maintained on free flow for 7–10 days.
- **Ureteric injury.** Call urologist; stent lumen or, if transected, end-to-end anastomosis (>6 cm from insertion into bladder) vs reimplantation into bladder (<6 cm from insertion into bladder).
- **Bowel injury.** Isolate with swabs to avoid leakage of bowel contents; call bowel surgeon; repair with fine (e.g. 3/0) absorbable sutures or bowel resection and anastomosis.
- **Vascular injury.** Call vascular surgeon: laparotomy (if laparoscopic injury); direct compression to control blood loss; use of atraumatic vascular clamps to occlude the injured vessel, avoiding intimai crush injury, blood/volume replacement; expose injury site; repair vessel wall with precise (intima-to-intima apposition); consider grafting depending upon extent of injury.

ENDOSCOPIC SURGERY

Endoscopic procedures

The three most common endoscopic techniques in gynaecology are as follows:

1. **Hysteroscopy** – Direct visualisation of the uterine cavity
2. **Cystoscopy** – Direct visualisation of the bladder
3. **Laparoscopy** – Direct visualisation of the peritoneal cavity

HYSTEROSCOPY

- **Technique**
  - Remove air bubbles.
  - Insertion with minimal distension pressure to optimise view.
  - Systematic inspection of uterine cavity (both tubal ostia, fundus, anterior/ posterior/side walls, isthmus, panoramic view of cavity and cervical canal).
- **Diagnostic indications**
  - Abnormal uterine bleeding
  - Infertility
  - Recurrent pregnancy loss
  - Abnormal glandular cervical smears
- **Common pathologies:** endometrial hyperplasia and cancer, polyps, fibroids, adhesions, congenital uterine anomalies.
- **Operative:** biopsy, polypectomy, myomectomy, uteroplasty, ablation/resection of endometrium, sterilisation, removal of foreign bodies within the genital tract.

CYSTOSCOPY

- **Technique**
  - Remove air bubbles.
  - Inspection of urethra and insertion into urethra/bladder.
  - Systematic inspection of bladder (neck, trigone, ureteric orifices interureteric ridge, bladder floor, side walls, bladder dome [air bubble]).
- **Diagnostic indications**
  - Urinary symptoms (urgency-frequency syndrome, painful bladder syndrome)
  - Suspected operative trauma
  - Suspected anatomical lesions
  - Haematuria
  - Staging for gynaecological malignancy
- **Common pathologies:** interstitial cystitis, diverticuli, calculi, foreign bodies, carcinoma.

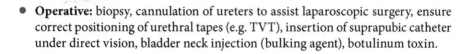

- **Operative:** biopsy, cannulation of ureters to assist laparoscopic surgery, ensure correct positioning of urethral tapes (e.g. TVT), insertion of suprapubic catheter under direct vision, bladder neck injection (bulking agent), botulinum toxin.

LAPAROSCOPY

- **Technique**
  - Dorso-lithotomy positioning of the patient (Trendelenburg; Lloyd-Davies).
  - 'Bottom end' – disinfect vagina, empty the urinary bladder, insert uterine manipulator (if applicable).
  - Establish pneumoperitoneum (insert the Veress needle vertically through a 1-cm intraumbilical incision; prior to insertion, the spring mechanism is checked on the needle to help avoid visceral puncture, and insufflator flow/ pressure is also checked).
  - Check intraperitoneal placement (drop test; high flow; low pressure).
  - Obtain sufficient pneumoperitoneum (25 mmHg).
  - Insert 10–12 mm umbilical trocar through the Veress needle incision (vertically with slight pelvic tilt).
  - Confirm entry into the peritoneal cavity (visualisation), lower the intra-abdominal pressure (15 mmHg), Trendelenburg position.
  - Systematic inspection of pelvis (uterus, adnexae, utero-vesical pouch, pouch of Douglas, uterosacral ligaments, peritoneal sidewalls, ovarian fossae, upper abdomen).
- **Diagnostic indications**
  - Infertility (adhesions – evidence of prior pelvic infection, congenital and acquired structural abnormalities of the uterus, endometriosis, Fallopian tube patency, feasibility of tubal reconstructive surgery)
  - Acute pelvic pain (acute pelvic inflammatory disease (PID), endometriosis, adnexal pathology/cystic accidents (haemorrhage, rupture, torsion), ectopic pregnancy
  - Appendicitis
  - Chronic pelvic pain (adhesions, endometriosis, chronic PID, adnexal pathology/cysts)
- **Common pathologies:** endometriosis, adhesions, pelvic infection, adnexal pathology (tubo-ovarian cysts, abscesses, masses, torsion, ectopic gestations).
- **Operative:** biopsy; tubal sterilisation, resection/ablation of endometriosis, ovarian cystectomy/oophorectomy, salpingectomy, myomectomy, hysterectomy.

Example descriptions of surgical instruments: key features of endoscopic equipment

Hysteroscopes

- Telescope (rigid or flexible) and diameter
- Proximal eye piece

- Angle of distal lens – usually 0°, 25°, 30° (look at the tip to see whether the lens is offset or look along the barrel of the scope as the distal lens angle is often inscribed along with the surgical manufacturer's name and diameter of instrument)
- Light source attachment
- Inflow port + Luer's lock (single channel, diagnostic set up)
- Inflow and outflow (continuous flow, operative set up) ports
- Operative working channel

Cystoscopes

- Telescope (rigid or flexible) and diameter
- Angle of distal lens – usually 0°, 12°, 30°, 70°, 120°
- Outer sheath and diameter
- Obturator
- Bridge (locking mechanism to hold telescope within the sheath)
- Light source attachment
- Working channel (often two for ureteric cannulation)

Laparoscopes

- Telescope and diameter
- Angle of distal lens – usually 0° or 30°
- Light source attachment
- Ancillary instrumentation (including trocars, traumatic and atraumatic graspers, scissors, energy modalities – monopolar diathermy, bipolar diathermy, ultrasonic instruments, advanced electrosurgical instrumentation)

Describing endoscopic instrumentation

Basic endoscopic examination requires the following equipment:

- Endoscope (rod lens or fibre-optic) for direct visualisation within body cavity or hollow viscus
- High-intensity light source and cable to provide illumination
- Camera with coupling lens and cable to video monitor to transmit and magnify image
- Distension media (conductive or non-conductive) to distend a body cavity or hollow viscus
- Ancillary instruments to manipulate, biopsy and operate

SURGICAL INSTRUMENTS AND INTERVENTIONS

You may be asked about common operative procedures in O&G and the instrumentation used in them. To aid revision, we have provided summaries of the instruments and interventions you should be familiar with.

Surgical instruments

If asked to describe and/or assemble surgical instruments, then concentrate on the following key points:

- When presented with an instrument, handle it in a steady, systematic fashion and hold it/assemble it in the way it is intended to be used. When you are nervous, there is a tendency to manipulate the instrument excessively and this can give the impression that you lack familiarity with the equipment, so handle it in a purposeful but sparing fashion.
- Do not answer the examiner's questions immediately even if you are certain of the answer. Pause for a few seconds before answering to allow you to compose your thoughts and formulate an answer.
- You can state what the equipment is and then proceed to describe its key features or begin with the description and then state what it is and what you would use it for.

Instruments you should be prepared to describe

Gynaecology

- Basic surgical instruments, retractors and sutures
- Endoscopes + ancillary equipment

Obstetrics

- Basic surgical instruments, retractors and sutures
- Forceps and vacuum devices
- Foetal blood sampling equipment
- Tamponade balloons

Top tip!

Ask a scrub nurse/senior colleague to talk you through various pieces of equipment – names, key features, assembly and uses.

General surgical instruments used in O&G

Dissecting forceps (toothed and non-toothed)

Use: To handle tissue during dissection and suturing
Examples: Bonney, McIndoe, Gillies, DeBakey

Tissue forceps

Use: To handle tissue during dissection
Examples: Lanes, Littlewood, Allis, Green-Armitage, Babcock, Duval

Haemostatic 'artery' forceps

Use: To provide haemostasis by occluding bleeding points or small vascular pedicle
Examples: Mosquito, Spencer Wells, Kocher, Lahey

Hysterectomy clamps

Use: To secure vascular tissue pedicles at hysterectomy prior to mobilising and tying
Examples: Bonney, Heaney, Zeppelin, Moynihan, Lahey cholecystectomy

Abdominal hand-held retractors

Use: To expose the operating field
Examples: Langenbeck, Czerny, Morris, Doyen, Deaver, De Lee

Topics to prepare for discussion: instruments, design and function.

Obstetric procedures

Repair of episiotomy and tears

The objective is to provide haemostasis and approximate disrupted tissue to aid healing (do not apply excessive tension as this will induce ischaemia, pain and poor healing).

1. Adequate light and exposure, systematic inspection, regional or local anaesthesia (e.g. 1% lidocaine).
2. Appropriate suture material (Cochrane review recommends synthetic suture materials, e.g. polyglycolic acid or polyglactin, e.g. Vicryl Rapide® 2/0).
3. Leave small, non-bleeding lacerations to heal naturally by secondary intention.
4. Identify apex of tear, apply continuous locking or non-locking suture to appose edges of vaginal mucosa symmetrically without excessive tension (use anatomic landmarks to guide, e.g. hymenal ring, pigmentation of perineum).
5. Once the posterior vaginal fourchette is reached, the needle is passed through the mucosa to be brought out into the subcutaneous tissue of the perineal body, the first encountered perineal muscles approximated and the suture tied with the knot buried.
6. Use interrupted sutures to close remainder of torn muscles/tissues.
7. Close the perineal skin, starting at the distal apex with a continuous, subcutaneous suture and bury the knot at the proximal end.
8. Check for haemostasis, check adequacy of vaginal introitus with digital examination and perform gentle rectal examination with consent ± 100 mg diclofenac/1 g paracetamol suppository.

Alternative techniques include separate, continuous closure of deep and superficial perineal muscles; using the same continuous suture to close the skin.

Repair of third/fourth-degree tears

1. Perform in theatre with a regional anaesthetic (ensure adequate light, exposure, assistance and instruments).

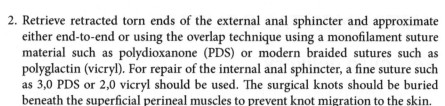

2. Retrieve retracted torn ends of the external anal sphincter and approximate either end-to-end or using the overlap technique using a monofilament suture material such as polydioxanone (PDS) or modern braided sutures such as polyglactin (vicryl). For repair of the internal anal sphincter, a fine suture such as 3,0 PDS or 2,0 vicryl should be used. The surgical knots should be buried beneath the superficial perineal muscles to prevent knot migration to the skin.

3. Use intraoperative and post-operative broad-spectrum antibiotics (e.g. co-amoxiclav/cephalexin + metronidazole) and laxatives (e.g. lactulose). All women should be offered physiotherapy and pelvic floor exercises and should be followed up (preferably in a specialist perineal trauma clinic). If a woman is experiencing pain or incontinence at follow-up, referral to a specialist gynaecologist or colorectal surgeon should be considered.

Topics to prepare for discussion: indications for episiotomy, definition of tears, causation, long-term complications, mode of subsequent delivery if third/fourth-degree tear.

FETAL BLOOD SAMPLING

1. Position patient (left lateral preferable to lithotomy) and prepare instrument tray.
2. Insert amnioscope appropriate to degree of cervical dilatation to approximate baby's scalp, withdraw introducer and attach light source.
3. Clean fetal scalp, spray with ethyl chloride (reactive hyperaemia) and apply Vaseline with a dental roll (surface tension).
4. Incise fetal scalp with a guarded blade at slight angle, wait for formation of blood droplet, apply capillary tube and collect blood.
5. Consider second sample whilst first is being analysed. Apply pressure with cotton wool ball to ensure haemostasis.

Topics to prepare for discussion: indications and contraindications, interpretation of results.

CERVICAL CERCLAGE

This technique is learnt as part of an advanced training study module in labour ward management, so you are unlikely to be asked specifically about it. However, be aware of the different techniques:

* Vaginal cerclage
  * McDonald suture
  * Shirodkar suture (vaginal incision, suture placed higher compared to McDonald suture)
* Abdominal cerclage (including laparoscopic)

Topics to prepare for discussion: indications, emergency cerclage.

INSTRUMENTAL DELIVERY

Ventouse delivery

1. Thorough abdominal/pelvic examination with particular attention to position and station of head.
2. Adequate analgesia/anaesthesia (perineal, pudendal, regional).
3. Empty the bladder (do not leave indwelling catheter).
4. Place cup as near as possible to posterior fontanelle (i.e. over flexing point of occiput).
5. Activate vacuum (negative pressure initially of 0.2 kg/cm^2, check cup position and exclude incorporation of vaginal mucosa, then increase to 0.8 kg/cm^2).
6. Apply traction synchronised with maternal contractions/expulsive efforts in the plane of the birth canal (i.e. the direction of pull will change as the head descends –downward – horizontal – vertical). Maximum of three pulls recommended.
7. Support and protect the perineum with non-dominant hand as head crowns and guide mother's expulsive efforts to ensure slow, gentle delivery with minimal trauma.
8. Carefully remove the Ventouse cup after switching off vacuum.

TRACTION FORCEPS DELIVERY

1. Thorough abdominal/pelvic examination with particular attention to position and station of head. Ensure that the sagittal suture is in the vertical plane.
2. Adequate analgesia/anaesthesia (perineal + pudendal, regional).
3. Assemble forceps to ensure correct type and they represent a 'set'.
4. Insert left blade with left hand, using right hand to guide and protect vagina. Repeat for right blade, this time using the opposite hand and bring the handles gently together to ensure easy locking in a horizontal plane with the sagittal suture remaining in a vertical plane.
5. Apply traction synchronised with maternal contractions/expulsive efforts in the plane of the birth canal (i.e. the direction of pull will change as the head descends – downward – horizontal – vertical). Maximum of three pulls recommended.
6. Make a right mediolateral episiotomy as the perineum is being stretched, support/ protect the perineum with non-dominant hand as head crowns and guide mother's expulsive efforts to ensure slow, gentle delivery with minimal trauma.
7. Carefully remove forceps blades.

Topics to prepare for discussion: relevant obstetric definitions (i.e. pelvic diameters, relationship of presenting part to pelvis, level of instrumental delivery), conditions required for safe application of instruments, indications and contraindications, change of instruments, trial of instrumental delivery, rotational delivery – manual, Ventouse and Kielland's forceps, complications.

CAESAREAN SECTION

Abdominal entry

1. Transverse, approximately 15 cm, symmetrical lower abdominal incision (Pfannenstiel or Cohen), approximately 2 cm above the symphysis pubis (below the superior aspect of the pubic hairline ideally).
2. Incise centrally through the subcutaneous tissues and rectus sheath followed by sharp or blunt extension of incision.
3. Parietal peritoneum identified between rectus muscles, peritoneum incised and opened in a transverse plane.
4. Uterine rotation corrected manually, insert Doyen retractor and expose lower part of the uterus.
5. Elevate uterovesical peritoneum, incise transversely using scissors and push lower edge of peritoneum and attached bladder inferiorly.

Uterine entry and delivery

1. Curved 3-cm incision into the now exposed lower uterine segment, careful entry into the uterine cavity using sharp or blunt dissection, membranes incised and fingers used bluntly to extend the incision laterally.
2. Insert hand inferiorly into the uterine cavity below the presenting part and gently elevate until presenting part appears within the uterine incision.
3. Fundal pressure applied by assistant and baby delivered.
4. Intravenous oxytocin administered by anaesthetist, placenta/membranes delivered with controlled cord traction and uterine cavity swabbed to remove any retained products of conception.

Surgical closure*

1. Closure of rectus sheath with continuous absorbable/non-absorbable suture (e.g. 1 Vicryl® or 1 Polydioxanone [PDS®]).
2. Skin closure with fine (e.g. 2/0) absorbable (e.g. Vicryl Rapide® or Monocryl®) or non-absorbable (e.g. 2/0 Proline®) subcutaneous suture.

*Peritoneal layers and fat layers do not require routine closure.

Topics to prepare for discussion: indications, classical uterine incisions, repeat caesarean sections, emergency second-stage operations, preterm delivery, oligohydramnios, abnormal lie, breech delivery, twin delivery, single versus double layer closure, high head/low head, placenta praevia, obesity, thromboprophylaxis, complications.

GYNAECOLOGICAL PROCEDURES

Vaginal hysterectomy

1. Incise and circumscribe the vaginal mucosa at the cervico-vaginal junction (most surgeons will empty the bladder and infiltrate the vaginal mucosa with saline/local anaesthetic and vasoconstrictors to reduce blood loss and help identify tissue plane).
2. Reflect the bladder from the cervix by sharp and/or blunt dissection.
3. Open the posterior peritoneum to enter the pouch of Douglas.
4. Clamp, cut and tie the uterosacral ligaments ± cardinal ligaments.
5. Open the anterior peritoneum to enter the utero-vesical space.
6. Clamp, cut and tie the uterine vessels within the broad ligament ± cardinal ligaments.
7. Deliver the uterine fundus into the vagina.
8. Clamp, cut and tie the ovarian ligament (infundibulo-pelvic ligament if salpingo-oophorectomy) and the round ligament.
9. Closure of vaginal vault, incorporating peritoneum and utero-sacral ligaments (for vault support). Commonly, a McCall culdoplasty is done (i.e. a single suture to incorporate the vaginal wall, peritoneum and utero-sacral ligaments, aimed at obliterating the posterior cul de sac).

Topic to prepare for discussion: contraindications.

Abdominal hysterectomy

There are many variations to the standard approach described as follows:

1. Transverse suprapubic incision (alternatively midline abdominal incision) ~2–3 cm above the symphysis pubis (below the superior aspect of the pubic hairline ideally).
2. Incise centrally through the subcutaneous tissues and rectus sheath and expose the underlying parietal peritoneum by incising the median raphe (pyrimidalis, if present, is reflected away at this point) followed by sharp or blunt extension of incision (± reflection of the rectus sheath of the underlying muscles in a cephalad direction if greater access required).
3. Parietal peritoneum identified between rectus muscles, peritoneum incised and opened in a transverse plane.

Hysterectomy

1. Place patient in Trendelenberg position, pack away bowel and insert self-retaining retractor.
2. Uterus stabilised, round ligament clamped and cut to enter the broad ligament (ureters can be identified retroperitoneally by further dissection through the areolar tissue into the base of the broad ligament).

3. Incise the posterior leaf of the broad ligament (after identifying the ureter intra- or extra-peritoneally), clamp and transect the ovarian ligament/Fallopian tube pedicle (infunidbulo-pelvic ligament if salpingo-oophorectomy) and ligate pedicle followed by round ligament. Repeat on the other side.
4. Reflect the bladder inferiorly by incising and dissecting the anterior leaf of the broad ligament and peritoneum of the utero-vesical fold.
5. Clamp, cut and tie the uterine vessels (if subtotal hysterectomy, transect uterus below these pedicles, cauterise the cervical canal ± oversew the supravagianl cervix).
6. Clamp, cut and tie the cardinal ligaments ± uterosacral ligaments.
7. Clamp vaginal angles, transect vagina and remove uterus (alternatively enter vagina centrally first, followed by clamping and transaction of the vaginal angles). Tie vaginal angles and close vagina (continuous or interrupted sutures – alternatively leave open using a purse-string vaginal suture).

Surgical closure*

1. Closure of rectus sheath with continuous absorbable/non-absorbable suture (e.g. 1 Vicryl® or 1 Polydioxanone [PDS®]).
2. Skin closure with fine (e.g. 2/0) absorbable (e.g. Vicryl Rapide® or Monocryl®) or non-absorbable (e.g. 2/0 Proline®) subcutaneous suture.

Total laparoscopic approaches to hysterectomy are becoming increasingly common. The operative steps are generally as described for abdominal hysterectomy. Dissection and ligation/cutting of tissue and vascular pedicles is achieved with electrosurgical or ultrasonic energy modalities. The operation is made easier by the use of specialised vaginal manipulators/cervical delineators which enhance surgical access and minimise the amount of tissue dissection required. The use of self-locking 'barbed' sutures further simplifies the procedure by avoiding the need for time-consuming knot tying.

Topics to prepare for discussion: route of hysterectomy (abdominal, laparoscopic, vaginal), total versus subtotal hysterectomy, complications.

EMERGENCY GYNAECOLOGICAL PROCEDURES

Evacuation of retained products of conception (surgical management of miscarriage)

1. Grasp the cervix with a vulsellum, ask the anaesthetist to administer 5 units of intravenous oxytocin and gently dilate the cervix using graduated Hegar dilators. If performing a manual vacuum aspiration (MVA) in a conscious

---

* Peritoneal layers and fat layers do not require routine closure.

woman, then administer direct cervical or paracervical local anaesthesia prior to cervical dilatation.

2. Insert suction cannula (e.g. Karman®, Ipas MVA Plus®) of appropriate diameter to the uterine fundus and evacuate the uterine cavity using gentle rotatory and back-and-forth movements (an empty cavity is suggested by uterine contraction and 'gritty' sensation as the suction catheter abrades uterine walls. Gentle blunt curettage can be used to confirm that the cavity is empty).

3. Alternatively, a blunt curette and/or polyp forceps can be used to retrieve the products of conception.

Topics to prepare for discussion: cervical prostaglandin preparation, role of antibiotics/genital tract screening, indications/contraindications for surgical management of miscarriage, surgical ERPC for trophoblastic disease.

Bartholin's abscess (incision and drainage)

1. Open (linear incision should be made over the medial pointing surface), drain and send pus to microbiology. Drainage should be ensured by the insertion of a gauze wick.

2. Consider treatment with appropriate antibiotics if the patient is febrile, the abscess large or there is surrounding cellulitis (the most common organisms are streptococci, *Escherichia coli*, proteus, chlamydia and gonococci).

3. Marsupialisation involves incising and draining the abscess followed by suturing the edge of the infected cyst cavity to the labial skin edges using interrupted, dissolvable sutures to lay it open, reducing the chance of recurrence.

4. Use of a short-stem balloon (Word) catheter is an alternative outpatient approach with a similar recurrence risk. After applying topical and/or injected local anaesthesia, a small stab incision is made to drain the lesion, saline lavage applied and the balloon catheter inserted and inflated with 2–5 mL of saline, which allows the catheter to remain in the cyst or abscess cavity for up to 4 weeks to allow epithelialisation of the tract at which point the catheter is deflated and removed if it has not been spontaneously expelled.

Ectopic pregnancy

1. **Salpingectomy.** The Fallopian tube containing the ectopic gestation is identified, elevated, separated from the ovary and removed by cutting and ligating the mesosalpinx and tube proximal to the products of conception. This is preferably achieved laparoscopically (using preformed 'endoloops' or energy modalities such as electrodiathermy) as surgical morbidity and the recovery time is reduced compared to laparotomy (suprapubic or midline incision).

   A partial salpingectomy removes a short section of tube containing the ectopic rather than the whole length of tube.

2. **Salpingotomy.** This involves a linear incision along the antimesenteric border of the tube over the ectopic gestation, the products of conception are removed

mechanically or with suction and the bleeding points are coagulated. This technique should be reserved for managing tubal pregnancy in the presence of contralateral tubal disease and the desire for future fertility.

Topics to prepare for discussion: advantages/disadvantages of salpingectomy versus salpingotomy, when to perform laparotomy.

EXAMPLE STRUCTURE ORAL EXAMINATION

Candidate's instructions

At this station, you will have 10 minutes to answer structured questions. The examiner will ask you a series of questions about the practice of operative vaginal delivery and will provide you with relevant instruments as part of the structured oral examination, which will assess the following domains:

- Communication with colleagues
- Applied clinical knowledge
- Patient safety

Examiner's instructions

This is a structured oral examination and assessment of practical skills. At this station, the candidate will have 10 minutes to answer questions related to endoscopic surgery and demonstrate the relevant competencies. You should ask the candidate the questions provided and give the ventouse devices and pelvic/fetal model to the candidate as appropriate. You can prompt the candidate if necessary, but this requirement should be reflected in the marks awarded.

You should have the following equipment:

- Silicone rubber cup (Silastic cup)
- Kiwi™ OmniCup (Bird modification cup)
- Pelvic model
- 'Fetal' doll

Questions to be asked:

Give the candidate the two ventouse vacuum devices (Figure 6.1).

1. Ask the candidate to identify each instrument and to describe the key design differences between the devices? Then ask what fetal position and type of operative delivery they would use each device for.
2. Assuming the prerequisites for operative vaginal delivery have been satisfied, what are the specific contra-indications for use of ventouse-assisted vaginal delivery?

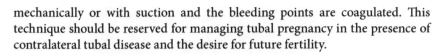

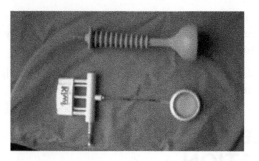

Figure 6.1 Ventouse vacuum devices.

Give the candidate the Kiwi OmniCup (Bird) and hold the model of the female pelvis and baby. Hold the doll in an occipito-posterior (OP) position.

3. Ask the candidate to describe and show you the optimal placement of the ventouse cup.
4. When would you abandon ventouse operative vaginal delivery?
5. If the ventouse fails, when would you apply obstetric forceps and what would you do before applying them?

MARKING

Communication with colleagues

- Clearly explains clinical concepts.
- Applies a structured approach during the discussion about using a second instrument.
- Seeks senior assistance when appropriate

Applied clinical knowledge

- Demonstrates the optimal placement for a ventouse cup.
- Identifies the instruments and shows an understanding of the fetal position and type of operative delivery they would use each device for.
- Is aware of when and if to consider a second instrument.

Patient safety

- Knowledge of the contraindications of ventouse delivery.
- Is aware of the reasons to abandon a ventouse cup delivery.
- Gives considered reasons for when to try a second instrument.

EXAMINER NOTES

1. **Ask the candidate to identify each instrument and to describe the key design differences between the devices? Then ask what fetal position and type of operative delivery they would use each device for.**
   - Both ventouse devices – one silicone rubber cup and the other Kiwi™ OmniCup (Bird modification cup).
   - The Kiwi™ OmniCup
     - Modified Bird cup (low profile mushroom-shaped cup)
     - Traction + integral vacuum delivery system (foam filter, palm pump, vacuum indicator gauge and release button)
     - Sterile single use (disposable) device
   - Silicone rubber cup (Silastic-cup)
     - Bell-shaped soft flexible silicone rubber cup
     - Integrated vacuum (interior is lined with small projections to enable air to be evacuated) and traction shaft with moulded ridges to facilitate grip + need external suction device
     - Reusable (autoclavable)
   - Position/type of delivery
     - The Kiwi™ OmniCup (modified Bird cup): all OA, OT and OP fetal malpositions
     - Silicone rubber cup (Silastic-cup): OA position and outlet (vertex) deliveries
2. **Assuming the prerequisites for operative vaginal delivery have been satisfied, what are the specific contraindications for use of ventouse-assisted vaginal delivery?**
   - Face presentation
   - Marked active bleeding from a fetal blood sampling site
   - Gestation <34 weeks
3. **Ask the candidate to describe and show you the optimal placement of the ventouse cup.**
   Midline over the occiput covering the posterior fontanelle (middle of cup over the flexion point of the fetal head [3 cm forward of posterior fontanelle]).
4. **When would you abandon ventouse operative vaginal delivery?**
   - No evidence of progressive decent with each pull (the head, not just the scalp, should descend with each pull).
   - Delivery not imminent following three pulls/contractions (of a correctly applied instrument by an experienced operator).
   - >15 minutes elapsed since application of instrument.
   - More than one cup detachment (an experienced operator should be summoned after one detachment for reapplication if feasible).
   - Woman withdraws consent.
5. **If the ventouse fails, when would you apply obstetric forceps and what would you do before applying them?**
   - Prior to application
     - Explain situation to patient/couple.

- Call for help if senior help available and feasible.
- Re-examine the patient to recheck fetal position, station (is the head engaged? i.e. is the caput felt below the ischial spines?).
- Checks for signs of fetal distress (CTG, FHR) – if present reconsider.
- Careful reflection (only use sequential forceps judiciously, avoid if possible, abandon if not straightforward application or descent with one pull of forceps).
- Only use sequential obstetric forceps when failure with the ventouse occurs because of inadequate traction/vacuum. Specifically,
  - Consider following failure to gain adequate suction due to excessive caput or leaking equipment in a baby presenting by the vertex below the ischial spines.
  - Consider following cup detachment and failure to gain adequate suction on reapplication of cup after progressive decent with ventouse and fetal head (not caput) visible without parting the labia (outlet delivery).
  - Consider following incorrect placement of ventouse cup by an inexperienced operator which explains failure.

CHAPTER 7
EMERGENCIES

The ability to manage emergency situations is integral to the competent practice of O&G. Medical emergencies can be stressful at the best of times, but this is particularly true in the field of obstetrics where most acute, life-threatening events tend to occur. This is because in obstetrics, you are generally dealing with young, otherwise healthy women and their babies. The MRCOG Part 3 allows examiners to evaluate the ability of candidates to think clearly and act appropriately in the acute situation where the life of the mother or baby may be at stake. For the purpose of the Part 3 examination, we would recommend preparing and practicing commonly encountered emergency situations, in simulated 'emergency drills' if possible. There are some excellent postgraduate courses, e.g. the PRactical Obstetric MultiProfessional Training (PROMPT) course, in which attendance would be ideal preparation and give confidence to the Part 3 candidate. This chapter gives guidance on how to tackle these stations successfully and provides suggested summaries for revising. The management of less common obstetric emergencies, medical emergencies and trauma is beyond the scope of this revision book.

Emergency drills should be normal part of your O&G practice. Not only performing them but also teaching them. Emergency scenarios provide an ideal opportunity to test your teaching skills and you should also prepare to teach the emergency scenarios to a colleague. See chapter for details on teaching.

HOW TO APPROACH THE 'EMERGENCY' STATION

Digest the question/scenario before answering

Your aim is to not only to provide the correct information but also to do so in a logical, systematic manner to demonstrate confidence in your abilities to the examiner(s). This is unlikely to be achieved by the nervous, impetuous candidate who 'rushes in' with an answer without allowing due time for reflection.

Adopt a structured approach

You will normally be presented with a brief clinical scenario but to aid your initial rapid clinical assessment, do not forget to seek further important information from the midwife (and patient if appropriate) if the underlying clinical situation is unclear. Appropriate questioning will obviously depend upon the particular clinical scenario but may include questions such as: 'Does the patient have any medical problems?' (in the case of unexplained collapse); 'What is the estimated blood loss?' or 'Is the placenta low lying?' (in the case of haemorrhage); 'Have there been any antenatal problems?' (in the case of foetal distress). Such questioning should however take place simultaneously with ABC resuscitation: i.e. Airway, Breathing and ventilation, and Circulation, with aggressive volume replacement and control of haemorrhage (if present). Make a decision at this point about the need to 'call for help', which means having additional staff immediately available on the labour ward, as well as informing or acquiring senior (consultant) input.

ABC resuscitation

- Involve the anaesthetist to manage the airway, breathing (supplementary oxygen, e.g. 8 L/min) and ventilation.
- Manage the circulation with a minimum of two large-calibre intravenous lines (e.g. 16 gauge upwards).
- Take blood, which generally means a FBC, coagulation screen, U&Es and cross-match in the case of haemorrhage. In the case of unexplained collapse/altered consciousness, take a blood glucose, urates, LFTs and pregnancy test as appropriate.
- Replace circulating volume rapidly if blood loss suspected, using warmed crystalloid/colloid initially and blood/blood products when available.
- Monitoring (insert urinary catheter with hourly bag; continuous pulse/BP/ECG/oximeter monitoring; consider arterial/CVP lines).
- Stop the bleeding (approach depends upon the cause – see specific scenario summaries).

*O negative blood can be acquired immediately in acute haemorrhage with cardiovascular compromise or, if the blood group is known, then type-specific blood ordered (available in <10 minutes) in addition to a request for fully cross-matched blood.

If the scenario is an antenatal/perinatal obstetric emergency, then once maternal resuscitation has begun, assess the well-being and viability of the foetus (i.e. electronic foetal monitoring ± ultrasound if available). Clearly, if the scenario is one of foetal distress in an otherwise well mother, then ABCs are not required and you should move directly to assessment of the foetus and diagnosing the cause of the foetal problem. Once resuscitation has begun (and the patient's condition is stabilising), then review the medical history and perform an abdominal/pelvic examination ± systemic examination as appropriate to arrive at a probable diagnosis (e.g. placental abruption, cord prolapse, pre-eclampsia/eclampsia). Finally, specific treatment should be instituted according to the diagnosis (e.g. uterotonic agents, antibiotics, delivery) and response to treatment evaluated on a continuous basis. Clear, contemporary documentation is key, both as a matter of good practice but also from the medicolegal standpoint. The overall approach is summarised in the box nearby.

Structured approach to managing emergencies in O&G

- Rapid assessment of situation + communicate
- ABC resuscitation
- Call for help (if appropriate)
- Assess foetal well-being and viability (if appropriate)
- Make a diagnosis
- Institute specific treatment
- Evaluation
- Documentation

Provide the information in the context of the real-life clinical setting

You will have encountered most situations in clinical practice. It is useful to 'picture' these past experiences in your mind to help assemble your thoughts in the correct sequence. Examiners will quickly spot the candidate who appears to be 'reciting from the textbook of obstetric emergencies' rather than relying on past clinical experience when describing their approach.

Remember to delegate and use facilities

The effective management of medical emergencies requires a multidisciplinary team approach. The question may 'provide' you with 'available staff', but, if not, it is reasonable to assume that you have resident midwives, healthcare assistants, porters, an SHO in obstetrics and an anaesthetic registrar, as well as available consultant staff in O&G, anaesthetics and haematology. In addition, most units have high dependency unit (HDU) beds on labour ward or available HDU/ITU beds elsewhere in the hospital. The good candidate will effectively delegate tasks according to experience and clinical competencies (see Chapter 9).

EMERGENCY SUMMARIES – OBSTETRIC EMERGENCIES

Pre-eclampsia/eclampsia

- Communicate.
- ABC (± CVP/arterial lines) and displacement of the uterus.
- Diagnosis (examination, FBC, U&Es, urate, coagulation screen, G&S, MSU).
- Control seizures (4 g $MgSO_4$ loading dose followed by 1 g/hour $MgSO_4$).
- Control hypertension (IV labetalol or hydralazine).

- Monitoring of blood pressure.
- Deliver.

Group specific or O rhesus negative

- Blood loss greater than 1000 mL.
- Communicate.
- ABC (± CVP/arterial lines) including Oxygen (15 L).
- Replace circulating volume (e.g. 2 L isotonic crystalloid, 1.5 L colloid).
- Blood (group specific of O rhesus negative).
- Blood products (platelets, cryoprecipitate, factor VIIa, fresh frozen plasma).
- Diagnosis (examination, FBC ± Kleihauer, coagulation screen, cross-match).
- Stop bleeding.

Uterine atony

- Bimanual compression and rub up the uterine fundus.
- Empty bladder.
- Uterotonic agents: Oxytocin (5 IU); Ergometrine (500 mg IV or IM); Oxytocin infusion (40IU in 500 mL); Carboprost (0.25 mg IM, every 15 minutes up to 8 times); Carboprost (intramyometrial 0.5 mg); Misoprostol (800 µg sublingually); Tranexamic acid (1 g IV).
- Examination under anaesthetic.
- Intrauterine balloon tamponade.
- Surgical management: brace suture, bilateral iliac ligation, hysterectomy.
- Uterine artery embolisation by interventional radiology.

Disseminated intravascular coagulopathy

Clotting factors (FFP/cryoprecipitate and platelets)

Genital tract trauma

- Repair of uterine/genital tract injury
- Topical fibrin

Signs of hypovolaemia

- Tachycardia
- Hypotension*
- Cold, clammy, pale skin (especially peripheries)
- Poor urine output
- Altered conscious level

*Hypotension (this is a relatively late sign associated with significant blood loss as the cardiovascular system in most young women will compensate initially, such that up to 35% of their circulating blood volume may be lost before the blood pressure falls).

Antepartum haemorrhage

- Communicate.
- Resuscitation as for 'massive obstetric haemorrhage' if major APH with haemodynamic shock.
- Diagnosis (examination – abdominal [abruption], speculum [local cause], USS to exclude placenta praevia [no VE unless this is excluded], FBC ± Kleihauer [give anti-D 500 IU if Rhesus negative], coagulation screen, cross-match).
- Assess foetal well-being.
- *Placental abruption.* Deliver foetus* (C/S vs IOL) if foetal or maternal compromise.
- *Placenta praevia.* Deliver foetus* (C/S) if foetal or maternal compromise.

*Threshold for delivery will depend upon gestation.

Uterine inversion

- Communicate.
- ABC (± CVP/arterial lines).
- Replace circulating volume/blood/blood products.
- Diagnosis (vaginal examination, FBC, coagulation screen, cross-match).
- Replace inversion as soon as possible (do not remove placenta until uterus is replaced):
    - Manual replacement
    - Hydrostatic repositioning (O'Sullivan's technique)
    - Consider uterine relaxation to facilitate (e.g. terbutaline, volatile agent [GA])
    - Surgical replacement (laparotomy)

Cord prolapse

- Communicate.
- Diagnosis (VE).
- Assess foetal well-being (EFM).
- Relieve pressure on umbilical cord:
    - Manual elevation + knee-chest or Trendelenburg positioning
    - Bladder filling (Foley catheter + 500 mL Normal saline)
    - Knee-to-chest position
    - Left lateral position with head down and a pillow under the left knee or hip
    - Consider tocolysis (terbutaline)
- Caesarean section or instrumental delivery, if fully dilated. The speed of delivery will depend on the foetal heart rate and the gestational age.

Shoulder dystocia

- Communicate.
- Position patient (draw buttocks to edge of bed; lie supine and hyperflex hips–McRobert's manoeuvre).

- Consider episiotomy.
- Suprapubic pressure + traction.
- Manoeuvres (deliver posterior arm/shoulder; internal rotatory manoeuvres, e.g. Woods' screw).
- Change of position (on all fours – Gaskin manoeuvre).
- Extreme measures (Zavanelli manoeuvre, cleidotomy; symphysiotomy).
- Examine genital tract for trauma and repair.

Twin pregnancy

- Inform anaesthetist/paediatrician/neonatal unit.
- Epidural can for useful due to potential uterine manipulations.
- Deliver twin I.
- Check lie (clinical/USS) and FHR twin II (EFM).
- Stabilise the second twin if it is cephalic, otherwise external cephalic version can be attempted. If this fails, then C/S, or internal podalic version with breech extraction, can be performed.
- ARM with contraction when presenting part is in the pelvis.
- Consider starting Oxytocin infusion to ensure contractions to not diminish.
- Aim for NVD (instrumental delivery if delay or foetal distress).
- Due to the increased risk of PPH, start post-natal Oxytocin infusion.

Vaginal breech delivery

- Consider epidural (potential need for vaginal manipulations).
- Await breech descent to pelvic floor before maternal pushing and await spontaneous delivery of breech +/– episiotomy (once anus visible over fourchette; note: 'hands off').
- Ensure sacrum rotates anteriorly using traction on the bony prominences of the hips.
- Delivery of extended hips can be achieved by flexion at the popliteal fossa.
- Avoid handling of the umbilical cord when manipulating the foetal body.
- Deliver anterior arm (once anterior shoulder scapula visible – run finger over shoulder to elbow and 'sweep' out by flexion and traction at elbow joint. Repeat for other (which will rotate anteriorly); Lovsett's manoeuvre for hyperextended/nuchal arm).
- Delivery of head
    - Consider suprapubic pressure to assist flexion of the head.
    - Mauriceau–Smellie–Veit manoeuvre: Once the occiput is visible, place two fingers on the malar prominences with the hand supporting the foetal body. The other hand presses on the foetal shoulders with the middle finger or fingers flex the occiput.
    - Burns Marshall manoeuvre: the foetal body is raised vertically to allow the head to be delivered spontaneously.
    - Forceps: if the head does not deliver, forceps can be used with the handles inserted underneath the foetal body and downward traction applied.

EMERGENCY SUMMARIES – GYNAECOLOGICAL EMERGENCIES

Miscarriage and haemorrhage with haemodynamic shock

- Communicate.
- ABC.
- Diagnosis (examination and remove products of conception from cervical canal [resolves vaso-vagal reaction], FBC, coagulation screen, G&S).
- Syntometrine® IM/IV (oxytocin 5 IU + ergometrine 0.5 mg).
- Transfer to theatre.
- Surgical ERPC.

Ruptured ectopic pregnancy with haemodynamic shock

- Communicate.
- ABC (± CVP/arterial lines – do not delay surgical intervention).
- Diagnosis (examination, urinary pregnancy test, FBC, coagulation screen, G&S).
- Transfer to theatre.
- Laparotomy.

EXAMPLE QUESTION AND STRUCTURED MARK SHEET

Shoulder dystocia (Practical competencies)

Candidate's instructions

At this station, you will have 10 minutes to answer questions and demonstrate practical competencies in relation to management of an obstetric emergency delivery. This station will assess the following domains:

- Patient safety
- Communication with colleagues
- Applied clinical knowledge

You are the registrar on call for obstetrics, and the emergency alarm sounds on the labour ward with an instruction to go to room 7 immediately. You arrive to find the baby's head has been delivered, but the midwife cannot deliver the shoulders.

The examiner will ask you to discuss and demonstrate, using the pelvis and provided, how you would manage the situation.

Marks will be awarded for

- Demonstrating practical skills and proficiency.
- Understanding of the manoeuvres available, this sequence and their rationale.
- Other knowledge relevant to this obstetric emergency.

Examiner's instructions

You should ask the candidate to demonstrate the relevant manoeuvres in the management of this obstetric emergency and then ask the questions in the order they appear on your instruction sheet. You can prompt the candidate if necessary, but this requirement should be reflected in the marks awarded.

You should have the following equipment:

- 'Foetal' doll
- Pelvic model

Questions to be asked:

1. Ask the candidate to take you through the steps in managing this obstetric emergency and demonstrate the relevant obstetric manoeuvres in a logical sequence using the doll provided. You should hold the pelvis as required.
   Once the candidate has finished, ask them the following questions.
2. How does shoulder dystocia happen?
3. What factors may be associated with shoulder dystocia?
4. What pre-emptive action to prevent shoulder dystocia would you consider in a diabetic woman with a BMI of 35 and a 4.3 kg baby?

MARKING SCHEME

Patient safety

- Appropriate prioritisation throughout.
- Calls for help.
- Does not apply fundal pressure and stops maternal pushing until shoulder displacement has been achieved.
- Appreciates that an experienced obstetrician should be available during delivery when there is a high risk of shoulder dystocia.

Communication with colleagues

- Describes how they would delegate tasks to colleagues and midwives.
- Ability to describe a clear action plan and rationale for the decisions made based on the discussions with the examiner.
- Communicates their management plan clearly.

Applied clinical knowledge

- Knows the correct sequence of steps for shoulder dystocia management.
- Understands the mechanism of action and the risk factors for shoulder dystocia.

EXAMINER NOTES ON SHOULDER DYSTOCIA

1. **Ask the candidate to take you through the steps in managing this obstetric emergency and demonstrate the relevant obstetric manoeuvres in a logical sequence using the doll provided.**
   - Call for help. Expertise is important – senior obstetrician, midwives/ancillary staff, anaesthetist, paediatrician (SpR upwards). Minutes count in baby's prognosis if asphyxia/trauma.
   - Take bottom of the bed and draw the buttocks to the edge. This allows optimal lateral flexion.
   - Consider episiotomy:
     - Allows room for internal manoeuvres (access to sacral hollow).
     - Reduce likelihood of vaginal lacerations.
   - McRobert's manoeuvre – maximum flexion, abduction and external rotation of the hips (manual, not lithotomy poles) ± moderate traction. This straightens the sacrum relative to the lumbar vertebrae, leading to upward rotation of the pelvis, freeing the impacted shoulder + also increases the uterine pressure and amplitude of contractions.
   - Suprapubic pressure + moderate traction – heel of hand applies constant or rocking pressure (for 30 seconds) (in a downward and lateral direction) to the posterior aspect of the shoulder. This adducts, reducing the bisacromial diameter, and internally rotates the anterior shoulder into the oblique pelvic diameter; it should then slip underneath the symphysis pubis with the aid of routine traction.
   - Deliver posterior arm and shoulder – operator's hand is passed up to the foetal axilla, gentle traction applied posteriorly and the shoulder hooked down bringing the posterior arm into reach. Then apply backward pressure on the cubital fossa to disimpact the arm. Hold the foetal hand and sweep it across the chest and face and out of the vagina:
     - More room in sacral hollow (thus go for posterior shoulder).
     - Access the shoulder and disengage the foetal arm to enable delivery.
   - Internal rotational manoeuvres: aim is to rotate the shoulders into an oblique diameter or by a full 180°:
     1. Wood's screw – Insert the fingers of the opposite hand vaginally so that you approach the posterior shoulder from the front of the foetus, aiming to rotate the shoulder towards the symphysis pubis.
     2. Reverse screw – Place fingers on the posterior shoulder from behind the foetus and rotate in the opposite direction.

3. Rubin II – Insert the fingertips behind the anterior shoulder and push it forward towards the foetal chest (adducting the shoulders and rotating the bisacromial diameter into the oblique). This manoeuvre can be combined with the Wood's screw to rotate the shoulders through 180°.

- Change of position – Roll over onto all fours ('Gaskin' manoeuvre). This increases the AP diameter of the inlet and facilitates other manoeuvres (e.g. delivery of posterior with respect to the maternal pelvis) shoulder.
- Extreme measures:
  - Zavanelli manoeuvre (cephalic replacement by rotating/flexing/reinserting foetal head into the vagina followed by C/S). This bypasses pelvic outlet.
  - Symphysiotomy (incomplete midline cut through the cartilaginous symphyseal joint). This increases the space available to facilitate delivery of the shoulders.
  - Cleidotomy. This allows excess adduction and manipulation of the foetal shoulder and arm.
- Do not
  - Apply fundal pressure.
  - Encourage maternal pushing efforts unless shoulder displacement has been achieved.

  Once the candidate has finished, ask them the following questions.

2. How does shoulder dystocia happen?

Failure of the shoulders to rotate into the AP diameter as they traverse the pelvic cavity. The posterior shoulder usually enters the pelvic cavity while the anterior shoulder remains hooked behind the symphysis pubis. In more severe forms, both shoulders do cross the pelvic brim.

3. What factors may be associated with shoulder dystocia?

- Antenatal factors:
  - Previous shoulder dystocia
  - Macrosomia
  - Diabetes mellitus
  - Maternal BMI > 30 kg/m^2
  - Induction of labour
- Intrapartum factors:
  - Prolonged first stage of labour
  - Secondary arrest
  - Prolonged second stage of labour
  - Oxytocin augmentation
  - Assisted vaginal delivery

4. What pre-emptive action to prevent shoulder dystocia would you consider in a diabetic woman with a BMI of 35 and a 4.3 kg baby?

- Consider C/S or induction of labour.
- Experienced obstetrician (SpR upwards) should be available on labour ward during the second stage of labour.

CHAPTER 8
STRUCTURED ORAL EXAMINATION (VIVA)

The structured oral examination or viva is a station where you will be asked a set of ordered questions by the examiner. Many candidates will be familiar with viva examinations from their undergraduate days or job interviews. Even if you are not, the station format is straightforward and this form of oral exam allows you an opportunity to demonstrate your knowledge and ability to communicate. A suggested, successful approach to these stations is outlined below.

DEMEANOUR

- Greet and/or introduce yourself. Stay calm and be pleasant.
- Be attentive – This means maintain a good posture (do not slouch) and eye contact, and, despite your nerves, aim to look interested and smile!
- Stay focused throughout, maintain your self-confidence and composure even if you feel the interview is not going well.
- Do not become argumentative or allow the discussion to become heated, even if you feel the examiner is unreasonably critical.
- Do not be alarmed if the examiner finishes questioning you before the bell goes. You have probably done well. Simply sit quietly unless the examiner wants to engage you in conversation. Resist the temptation to ask: 'How have I done?'
- Thank the examiner when leaving the station.

ANSWERING QUESTIONS

Listen carefully to the question and answer directly. It is surprisingly common for candidates to answer a different, often unrelated question! Indeed, this tendency is not limited to exam candidates but also to trainees or medical students usually as a result of becoming 'flustered' when they are 'put on the spot' by senior colleagues in day-to-day clinical practice settings. To an examiner this can be very irritating, especially when they are trying to follow a prepared format. Another annoyance to examiners is the 'parrot-like' repetition of their questions out of habit.

Follow instructions exactly – if a short answer is requested, keep your answer short. If more detail is desired, give a longer response. Try to answer the question as it is posed, remembering that you are engaged in an academic conversation.

Do not interrupt the examiner. Wait until they finish the question before you start to answer. Indeed, a good approach is to pause briefly after each question is asked. This allows you to take a moment to compose yourself, formulate some thoughts and decide where to begin.

Do not answer questions with just a 'yes' or 'no'. It is difficult to explore a candidate's knowledge if they are somewhat monosyllabic. You should demonstrate your in-depth knowledge by expanding on your answer. When you do this, however, it is important to ensure that you have clearly answered the set question that you are confident of the additional, related information you are now providing and you remain concise. (i.e. do not bore the examiner with a prepared speech!) Stick to two or three key points or examples.

If you have not understood the question, seek clarification by asking the examiner to rephrase it, or alternatively give your interpretation and ask if that is what was meant. If you still do not understand the question, then it is better to admit it than to try and bluff. Do not 'ramble' if you have understood the question but do not know an answer. In such circumstances, ask for clarification if appropriate, but if you are sure you cannot answer the question then admit this, i.e. state directly that you do not know the answer. This allows the examiner to rephrase the question, which may help you formulate an answer or move to the next question where you may score marks rather than wasting time 'digging a deep hole' that you cannot climb out of!

Do not carry 'baggage'. Remember that each new question represents a new opportunity to gain marks, so put a previous bad question to the back of your mind. There will be plenty of time to ruminate about this later, once the exam is over, but it will not help you in the exam and indeed will have a detrimental effect.

Come across as an 'intelligent listener', i.e. you are more likely to convey a good impression if you appear attentive and interested in what the examiner has to say. This is especially important if you have failed to answer a question correctly, as your apparent willingness to learn from the examiner will be looked upon favourably.

Engage the examiner. Although the emphasis of these structured oral tests is on your providing answers similar to those on the examiner's structured mark sheet, when a viva is going well, the interaction with the examiner is often a two-way process involving you talking *and* listening and maybe even discussing issues and providing opinions. A *viva voce* examination, say when presenting a university thesis, will set out to interrogate the candidate and test the limits of their knowledge. In this professional examination, this is not the aim, so if the examiner goes 'off message' and starts asking more dynamic, difficult, open-ended questions, then do not panic. It is likely the examiner thinks you are a good candidate and they are filling the time and enjoying the interaction.

Learn when to 'stop talking'! If the examiner identifies an area of weakness, concede the point gracefully. However, in clinical medicine, there is often no absolutely 'right' or 'wrong' answer, so be prepared to justify your answer. If the examiner challenges your position, then reconsider your answer, but if you still believe that your initial response was a good one, then present your case firmly but in a courteous manner.

EXAMPLE STRUCTURED ORAL EXAMINATION – OBESITY AND PREGNANCY

Candidate's instructions

At this station, you will have 10 minutes to answer questions about obstetric care.

This is a structured viva. The examiner will ask you a series of questions about issues relating to the management of obese women in pregnancy. It will assess the following domains:

- Communication with colleagues
- Applied clinical knowledge
- Patient safety

Marking

Communication with colleagues

- Clearly explains clinical concepts.
- Structures the risks and complications associated with obesity and pregnancy.
- Explains the antenatal and intrapartum care considerations in a methodical manner.

Applied clinical knowledge

- Clear understanding of the risks and complications associated with obesity and pregnancy.
- Is aware of how to manage an obese obstetric patient during pregnancy.
- Demonstrates understanding of the intraoperative considerations for an obese obstetric patient.

Patient safety

- Implements a safe antenatal management plan for the patient.
- Demonstrates safe surgical considerations for caesarean delivery of an obese obstetric patient.

Examiner's instructions

This is a structured viva assessing the candidate's knowledge regarding the obstetric care of obese women. You should ask the candidate the questions provided in sequence. If required, you can prompt the candidate; however, this should be reflected in your overall assessment.

Structured viva questions

1. *How would you define obesity?*
   BMI > 30 kg/m² at first contact.

2. *Obesity is considered a risk factor for pregnancy. What obstetric complications are associated with obesity?*
   - Antenatal
     - Gestational diabetes
     - Hypertension, pre-eclampsia
     - Abnormal foetal growth: either macrosomia or IUGR
     - Sleep apnoea
     - Undiagnosed foetal anomaly
   - Intrapartum
     - Failure to progress in labour
     - Shoulder dystocia
     - Difficulties monitoring foetal heart
     - Inadequate analgesia
     - Emergency C/S
     - Technically difficult C/S, with associated increased morbidity and mortality
     - Anaesthetic risks
     - Other theatre risks – positioning/moving of the patient difficult, compromised safe use of equipment, such as lithotomy stirrups, operating tables
   - Postpartum
     - Wound infections post-operative delivery
     - Thromboembolic events
     - Postnatal depression

3. *What additional antenatal care would you arrange for a nulliparous 27-year-old woman with a BMI of 44 kg/m² who you are seeing at a booking antenatal clinic appointment?*
   - Consultant-led care if BMI > 35.
   - Glucose tolerance test (GTT) at 26 weeks to check the development of gestational diabetes.
   - Encourage healthy eating and offer an appointment with a dietitian.
   - Obstetric/medical risk factors related to the obesity (as outlined previously) need to be discussed with the woman and documented in a frank but sensitive way.
   - Low-dose aspirin (nulliparous + BMI >35 = two moderate risk factors for pre-eclampsia as per NICE guidance)
   - Consider USS scans for foetal growth ± well-being (foetal weight, liquor volume and umbilical artery Doppler studies) in the third trimester (e.g. 28–34 weeks) as it can be difficult to estimate growth from palpation alone in obese women.
   - Increase frequency of antenatal clinic appointments (hospital and community) due to the increased risk of pregnancy complications in this group of women (e.g. schedule at least 2 weekly from 28 weeks and weekly

from 36 weeks). Blood pressure should be checked with an appropriately sized cuff at each visit.

- Refer for an anaesthetic assessment regardless of the planned mode of delivery (e.g. between 28 and 34 weeks for most women) particularly to assess the safety of category 1 caesarean delivery versus elective delivery. The woman should be re-weighed (feasibility of obstetric operating tables, etc.).
- Arrange social service support, psychiatric input, etc., if social disadvantage, domestic violence, mental illness, etc., associated with obesity.

4. *This woman (BMI 44) requires an emergency C/S for a deep transverse arrest causing failure to progress in the second stage of labour. It is 02:00 and your consultant is at home. What intra- and post-operative problems would you anticipate and how would you minimise these?*
   - Difficulty with moving and positioning the patient. Ensure adequate staffing, appropriate weight-bearing equipment, e.g. operative table, extra assistance.
   - Difficult anaesthesia. Ensure Obstetric SpR has discussed the case with their on-call consultant and asked for assistance (two anaesthetists preferable) if deemed necessary (especially if they cannot gain regional access).
   - Difficult surgical access (fat patient cannot lie flat for anaesthesia). Extra assistance (ideally senior), large Pfannensteil incision (midline rarely required to access uterus but consider if other risk factors, e.g. adhesions from previous surgery), careful abdominal entry to ensure adequate access prior to incising the uterus.
   - Wound infection. Good surgical technique (careful tissue handling, haemostasis) and use interrupted skin sutures/staples (reduce collection/abscess). Use of broad-spectrum antibiotics intrapartum and consider postpartum. Regular review (daily).
   - Venous thromboembolism. Keep well hydrated, use of intraoperative pneumatic compression stockings, administer prophylactic postpartum anticoagulant, e.g. Dalteparin (Fragmin) 5,000 IU SC to upper thigh, every 24 hours (first dose to be administered no sooner than 4 hours postoperatively and no later than 24 hours postoperatively. Treatment is to be continued for a minimum of 4 days). Consider use of postpartum TED stockings.

5. *You have difficulty delivering the impacted foetal head. What do you do to aid delivery of the baby*
   Methods to facilitate extraction of the impacted head:
   - 'Push' method. Place patient in the Whitmore (frog) position and push the deeply engaged head upwards through the vagina out of the pelvis. This manoeuvre can be done by the operator or, more usually, an assistant.
   - 'Pull' method (reverse breech)
     - Introduce your hand through the LUS incision and up towards the upper segment, grasp the foetal legs and extract the foetus by the breech.
     - LUS transverse incision may need to be adapted into an inverted T or J incision.
     - ± Uterine relaxation (inhalational agent [GA]/β-mimetic, e.g. terbutaline).
     - Call consultant.

CHAPTER 9
TEACHING

It is inevitable that you will encounter a teaching station as part of your MRCOG Part 3 Task Circuit. A teaching station enables the examiner to assess several domains including patient safety, applied clinical knowledge and communication with colleagues.

Teaching is a component of all trainees work but just like a surgical procedure, it can be performed well or badly. Some trainees have a natural flare for teaching whilst others struggle to convey concepts or demonstrate practical skills. In this chapter, we have summarised the key issues in how to succeed in a teaching station, from the general approach to a step-by-step guide to be able to teach any form of knowledge or skill so that it may be adapted to any type of teaching task.

As with all of the other types of teaching station, it is imperative to understand the task at hand. The 2-minute reading time before the start of the station is of key importance in a teaching station. It allows you to formulate a strategy for your teaching that you can refer to in the 12-minute station.

APPROACHES TO A TEACHING STATION

Those of you that have a natural talent for teaching your junior colleagues or medical students are likely to adopt a structured approach to teaching without consciously deciding to do so. The aim of a teaching session is to provide a planned experience such that there is an improvement in knowledge or skills. Providing structure to this planned experience optimises the chance that there will be improvement. In general, there are three core components of any teaching event:

1. The environment
2. The teaching/demonstration
3. The summary

The environment

You may well have had personal experience of poor teaching environments before. A perfect example of a poor teaching environment would be all of those times that you have lost concentration and even fallen asleep (!) in a lecture theatre, because it was too warm or too crowded. For the learner to be engaged, the environment for the teaching event must be optimised to maximise learning. The environment includes heating, lighting, ventilation, acoustics and the arrangement of furniture.

Clearly, for the MRCOG Part 3 exam, you cannot make wholesale changes to the environment of the Task cubicle. However, you can still optimise the environment for your teaching event. The most likely scenario you will encounter in a teaching station is where you are prompted to teach a practical skill to a junior colleague or medical student. You can improve the environment for learning by doing some simple things. For example, you can help engagement and concentration by moving your chair closer to the learner's. Explain why you are doing this. Place props that you are provided with equidistantly between you and the learner so that they have the opportunity to also touch and feel the prop and see exactly what you are demonstrating. These may sound like simple suggestions, but we have always been amazed at the number of candidates who sit across the table from the candidate and hold the prop themselves and never pass the prop on to the learner.

The teaching/demonstration

Most medical educators would argue that the introduction to the teaching session is the most important part of the teaching event. The next time you are due to teach medical students, at the beginning of the lecture, state that the content of the lecture will appear in their end of year exam. You will witness the immediate uplift in motivation and engagement demonstrated by your students! The reason for this phenomenon is that the students now understand that the content of your teaching is highly useful to them (to pass their end of year exam). Clearly you should not say this in the MRCOG Part 3 exam, but motivating the learner to learn is a crucial part of any teaching event. For the purposes of the teaching station, motivation can be instilled by saying 'I am going to teach you XXX because it is an important skill to learn to be able to YYY'.

Clear objectives should be stated and the role of the learner should be defined. The learner needs to know whether they are to be active or passive, whether they should ask questions or participate in any other way. At the end of the introduction, it is essential that the learner understands what you will teach them and why it is important to them.

It is also important to build some rapport with the student that you are teaching in the teaching station. If the student is a junior colleague or a medical student, this can be achieved by simply asking their name. Ask what stage of training they are at or whether they are enjoying O&G. Rapport is important to engage the learner.

The actual teaching matter is delivered after setting the objectives.

The summary

The last part of any teaching event should be some form of closure. An adequate closure to the teaching is achieved where the learner is left satisfied with the experience, having fully comprehended what they have been taught. In general, questions should be invited from the learner. Once these questions have been answered, you should try and summarise what you have taught and then make it clear that the end of the teaching episode has been reached.

WHAT KINDS OF TEACHING STATIONS ARE LIKELY TO COME UP?

The most likely teaching stations to arise will include teaching a practical skill, teaching the management of emergency, teaching a non-technical task and teaching about a particular clinical condition.

Teaching a practical skill

Examples:

- Performing a ventouse or forceps delivery
- Performing a breech vaginal delivery
- Performing laparoscopic entry
- Fitting a ring or shelf pessary

This is probably the most common type of teaching station. Many medical educators promote a four-stage process for teaching practical skills:

1. Demonstrate the practical skill in real time with or without verbal commentary from the teacher.
2. Repeat demonstration, usually at a slower pace, with verbal commentary from the teacher, justifying the actions.
3. Repeat demonstration by the teacher with verbal commentary from the learner.
4. Repeat demonstration by the learner with verbal commentary from the learner.

In the midst of the MRCOG Part 3 exam circuit, you may not be able to get through the practical skill four times and teach factual knowledge surrounding the skill. However, with time limited, you should be able to get through steps 2 and 4. This would show the examiner that you are able to demonstrate and verbally explain what you are doing and that you understand the importance of learner engagement through their active participation.

A good tip when demonstrating a practical procedure is to try and imagine that you are in the delivery room or operating theatre so that you do not miss out any key steps.

Teaching the management of an emergency

Examples:

- Management of post-partum haemorrhage
- Management of an eclamptic fit

Teaching management of emergency situations should be carried out in a stepwise manner. In no other situations is a logical stepwise approach more important than in an emergency situation. However, you should still discuss the importance of the condition and its incidence before focusing on the ABC resuscitation management steps. Do not forget the aftercare of patients involved in emergencies, including where to nurse them, completion of incident forms and contemporaneous documentation.

Teaching a non-technical task

Example:

- Taking consent for an operation

Teaching a non-technical skill could be seen as easier than teaching a practical skill. However, it may be more difficult in practice as there will inevitably be less interaction from the learner. It is vitally important in these situations to ask the learner questions throughout the teaching process to promote and heighten the level of engagement. Without this, the station will be over very quickly and you will have struggled to demonstrate your skills as a teacher.

For the given example of teaching the taking of informed patient consent, the teacher can ask the learner what they know about the operation, what indications they know of for the operation and what risks the operation carries. It would also be appropriate to enquire about the learner's understanding of providing valid consent. Lastly, the learner could be asked what to do at the end of the consent procedure. This could include inviting questions, providing a patient copy of the consent form, appropriate documentation in the medical notes and ensuring confirmation of consent on the day of the operation (two-stage consent process).

Teaching about a particular clinical condition

Examples:

- Teaching about HELLP syndrome
- Teaching about infertility
- Teaching about labour

When teaching about a clinical condition, it is important to employ a structured approach. One should stress the importance of the condition by teaching the incidence of the condition. Then a logical way would be to talk about its symptoms and signs, investigations and management.

Whatever the type of station, try to teach in a systematic, logical manner and ensure that there is interaction between yourself and the learner. Avoid a situation where you talk for the entire 12 minutes with the learner simply listening passively. This is unlikely to impress the examiner and leads to a sufficient mark to pass the task.

Don't forget to check the learner's understanding throughout the contact. Asking questions regularly regarding what you have just taught is better than simply asking whether the learner understands what you have taught.

USE OF PROPS

It is very likely that you will be given some props to make use of in a teaching station. Make sure that the prop is used effectively. Do not just wave it around aimlessly. When you are not using the prop, leave it on the table, to reduce the level of distraction as you are teaching. Once it is time to make use of the prop, ensure that you are making full use of it. For example, when demonstrating forceps delivery, give the learner the forceps to feel and touch. Ask them to name the different parts of the forceps blade whilst they hold it.

GOOD PRACTICES IN TEACHING

A summary of the steps involved in forming a good approach to a teaching station is provided as follows:

1. Read the instructions for the Task Station carefully.
   - What are you to teach?
   - Who are you to teach?
2. Introduce yourself and build rapport.
   - What is your name?
   - What level of training are you in?
3. Set the environment.
   - Place yourself close to the learner.
   - Place props equidistant between you.
4. Explain to them what you will teach.
   - Why is the topic that you are teaching important for them?
   - What do they know about this topic already?
5. Explain what you expect from them during the teaching.
   - You wish for them to stop you and ask questions throughout.
   - You wish them to demonstrate the practical skill after you show them how it is done.
6. Deliver the teaching.
   - See sections above for different types of teaching stations
7. Close the teaching.
   - Invite questions
   - Summarise what you have taught

EXAMPLE TEACHING STATIONS

- How to manage shoulder dystocia
- How to gain safe closed laparoscopic access

Example teaching station I

Candidate's instructions

This station is with a simulated junior trainee and will assess the following domains:

- Communication with colleagues
- Information gathering
- Applied clinical knowledge
- Patient safety

A second-year trainee has come to you for some advice. They are worried as they will become a third-year trainee in a matter of months and they are yet to independently manage a shoulder dystocia. They want some advice regarding how best to manage this clinical scenario.

You have 10 minutes in which to teach safe management of shoulder dystocia. This should include the following:

- The risk factors for shoulder dystocia and how you may be able to prevent shoulder dystocia
- How to diagnose shoulder dystocia
- The techniques to safely manage shoulder dystocia and their rationale
- Complications that may ensue after the management of shoulder dystocia

Simulated trainee instructions

You are a second-year specialist trainee in O&G. You will progress to the third year of your training in 3 months time. You are aware that you will be expected to manage obstetric emergencies independently but are worried, as you are yet to manage a shoulder dystocia independently. You have gone through obstetric emergency skills drills training and know the manoeuvres that are needed to manage shoulder dystocia but wish to go over identification and management of shoulder dystocia with your senior colleague. In particular, although you can recall the manoeuvres, you would like your senior colleague to show you exactly how to perform them and their rationale. You have seen shoulder dystocia managed before but found it difficult to see exactly how a senior colleague performed the necessary manoeuvres.

You are receptive to advice but seek clarification if the candidate sounds unsure.

If not covered by the candidate, questions that you could ask include:

- What is shoulder dystocia?
- What are the risk factors for shoulder dystocia?
- How do you know when shoulder dystocia is occurring?
- If shoulder dystocia is identified, what should the immediate management be?
- How is McRobert's manoeuvre performed?
- How should suprapubic pressure be performed?
- How should the enter manoeuvres be performed?
- What do you do if the enter manoeuvres do not work?
- What are the subsequent complications that may occur after the successful management of shoulder dystocia?

Marking

Communication with colleagues

- Appropriate introduction and attempts to build rapport.
- Tries to gain an understanding of the learning needs of the junior trainee – what do they know, what do they want to know more about.
- Has a clear learning structure with use of structured lists and mnemonics.
- Demonstrates practical manoeuvres and then allows the junior trainee to show that they can also perform the manoeuvres whilst offering constructive feedback.
- Encourages active practical participation from the junior trainee.
- Encourages learning, discussion and questions with appropriate verbal and non-verbal communication throughout.

Information gathering

- Attempts to identify what the junior trainee already knows and their existing experience of shoulder dystocia.
- Confirms that the junior trainee is receptive to advice at regular intervals and checks that the learning needs of the trainee have been met at the end of the teaching event.

Applied clinical knowledge

- Is able to provide a structured way of remembering risk factors for shoulder. Does not just provide a disorganised list of risk factors. Demonstrates that there may be no risk factors in the majority of deliveries complicated by shoulder dystocia.
- Is able to demonstrate how to identify shoulder dystocia and what it is.
- Teaches and demonstrates the management of shoulder dystocia in a sequential manner to encourage learning.
- Encourages vigilance against post-partum haemorrhage and to identify perineal trauma.
- Gives appropriate feedback and develops a learning plan using knowledge of the curriculum and assessment tools.

Safety

- The candidate teaches the junior trainee the risk factors of shoulder dystocia so that they may be able to predict when it may occur.
- The candidate demonstrates that they are able to identify shoulder dystocia and calls for help by declaring an emergency (e.g. by pulling the emergency buzzer).
- The candidate should advise the sequential manoeuvres to perform once shoulder dystocia has been identified.
- The candidate understands the potential foetal and maternal complications of shoulder dystocia.
- The candidate ensures that contemporaneous notes are recorded and an incident form is completed.

Examiner notes on shoulder dystocia

- The candidate is provided with a model pelvis and a foetal doll and should make use of the props provided in their teaching.
- Shoulder dystocia is when the anterior shoulder of the foetus is obstructed from delivery by the superior border of the pubic symphysis after delivery of the head. It is a bony obstruction to the complete delivery of the foetus. It is an obstetric emergency, and there is significant neonatal morbidity (brachial plexus injury) and mortality associated if shoulder dystocia is not managed promptly.
- Shoulder dystocia occurs in upto 1% of vaginal deliveries.
- The vast majority of deliveries complicated by shoulder dystocia have no risk factors. However, if risk factors are present, they can be divided into antenatal and intrapartum risk factors.
- The antenatal risk factors are maternal obesity, maternal short stature, previous shoulder dystocia, diabetes mellitus and induction of labour.
- The intrapartum risk factors are prolonged first or second stages of labour, use of oxytocics and operative vaginal delivery.
- Diagnosis of shoulder dystocia is aided by having a high index of suspicion when risk factors are present, turtle sign and foetal facial flushing after delivery of the head.
- The sequential management of shoulder dystocia can be remembered by the pneumonic HELPERR and should be accompanied by routine traction.
  - H: Call for Help – By pulling emergency buzzer to summon the senior obstetrician, midwives, anaesthetist, paediatrician.
  - E: Episiotomy – Evaluate or extend episiotomy to allow enter manoeuvres and to reduce further vaginal or perineal trauma.
  - L: Elevate legs – McRoberts maneouvre (full supine position with hyperflexion, external rotation and abduction of hips and knees) allows straightening of the sacrum and upward rotation of the pelvis.
  - P: Apply suprapubic pressure – From the foetal back with a rocking pressure with the aim to reduce the bisacromial diameter, rotating the anterior shoulder into an oblique dimension.
  - E: Enter manoeuvres – Internal rotation of the anterior and posterior shoulders
  - R: Remove posterior arm (identification of the posterior forearm and hand with gentle delivery).
  - R: Roll on to all fours.
- More drastic manoeuvres are only to be performed if the HELPERR pneumonic has been unsuccessful and include: Zavanelli's manoeuvre, intentional fracture of the foetal clavicle and symphsiotomy.
- An incident form should be completed, contemporaneous notes should be recorded and the woman debriefed.

Example teaching station 2

Candidate's instructions

This station is with a simulated junior trainee and will assess the following domains:

- Communication with colleagues
- Information gathering
- Applied clinical knowledge
- Patient safety

A first-year trainee in O&G has approached you to teach them how to gain closed laparoscopic access with a veress needle and primary and secondary port insertion.

You have 10 minutes in which to teach safe laparoscopic entry using a veress needle followed by safe insertion of the primary and secondary trocars. Your teaching should include the following:

- How to select the site of veress needle insertion
- The techniques to safely insert the veress needle at the umbilicus
- Safety checks to ensure that the veress needle has been inserted into the correct intraperitoneal position
- Introductory, insufflation and operating veress needle pressures
- Safe introduction of primary and secondary laparoscopic ports

Simulated trainee instructions

You are a first-year specialist trainee in O&G. You are to attend your first elective gynaecology operating list tomorrow, which has a number of laparoscopies to perform. You have not attended any surgery courses yet and do not want to show that you have no knowledge regarding laparoscopies to your consultant. You have never seen a veress needle before.

You are receptive to advice but seek clarification if the candidate sounds unsure.

If not covered by the candidate, questions that you could ask include the following:

- How do we decide where to insert the veress needle?
- How can I safely insert the veress needle and reduce the risk of injury to the bowel and blood vessels?
- Are there any checks that I can perform to check that the veress needle has been inserted to the correct location?
- How do I insert the laparoscopic ports?

Marking

Communication with colleagues

- Appropriate introduction and attempts to build rapport.
- Tries to gain an understanding of the learning needs of the junior trainee – what do they know, what do they want to know more about.
- Adopts a clear learning structure.

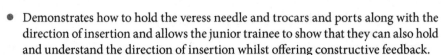

- Demonstrates how to hold the veress needle and trocars and ports along with the direction of insertion and allows the junior trainee to show that they can also hold and understand the direction of insertion whilst offering constructive feedback.
- Encourages active practical participation from the junior trainee.
- Encourages learning, discussion and questions with appropriate verbal and non-verbal communication throughout.

Information gathering

- Attempts to identify what the junior trainee already knows and their existing experience of laparoscopy.
- Checks understanding at regular intervals and checks that the learning needs of the trainee have been met at the end of the teaching event.

Applied clinical knowledge

- Provides a short list of contraindications to closed umbilical entry that the junior trainee should check for pre-operatively.
- Instructs the junior trainee to ensure that the patient is in a horizontal Lloyd-Davies position on the theatre table and to clean, drape and catheterise appropriately.
- Demonstrates clear understanding of safe closed veress needle entry at the umbilicus.
- Demonstrates clear knowledge of the safety checks to ensure correct veress needle positioning after insertion.
- Is able to teach the junior trainee the correct introductory, insufflation and maintenance operating pressures.
- Demonstrates safe techniques to introduce the laparoscopic ports.

Safety

- Understands the importance of safe veress needle entry.
- Understands the safety checks to ensure correct veress needle insertion.
- Demonstrates knowledge regarding safe entry pressures and pressures required to insert laparoscopic ports.
- Demonstrates a safe technique in laparoscopic port insertion.

Examiner notes on safe laparoscopic entry

- The candidate is provided with a veress needle, a 10 mm primary port and trocar and a 5 mm secondary port and trocar. The candidate should employ the props that are provided.
- Umbilical veress needle insertion should be avoided in women with low BMIs or in those who have had multiple previous lower transverse abdominal incisions or previous midline laparotomy. In these circumstances, entry at Palmer's point should be considered.
- The woman should be placed on a flat operating table (not Trendelenburg's) and the legs should be placed in the Lloyd-Davies position.

- The vagina should be cleaned, draped and the urinary bladder emptied. The uterine manipulator should be inserted.
- The abdomen should be cleaned and draped and examined to ensure there are no abdominal masses.
- The spring action of the veress needle should be checked, and the pressure and flow should be checked with the needle connected to a functioning insufflator.
- A 1 cm intraumbilical vertical incision should be made.
- The veress needle should be inserted in a vertical direction. There should be two clicks – from the fascia and the peritoneum. There should be no excessive lateral movements after insertion of the needle, which could exacerbate a bowel injury. Palmer's test (aspiration, injection and aspiration of saline through the veress needle) should be performed.
- Introductory pressure should be <8 mmHg and there should be high flow of carbon dioxide in to the abdomen.
- The abdomen should be insufflated to 25 mmHg to form a tense pneumoperitoneum.
- A two-hand screwing technique should be used to insert the primary trocar at a 90° angle to the skin. The trocar should be removed as soon as it has entered the abdominal cavity.
- The laparoscope should be inserted immediately and a 360° survey of the abdominal cavity should be performed to check for adherent bowel.
- A 5 mm incision should be made lateral to the inferior epigastric artery with transillumination to ensure that in abdominal wall no vessel is damaged. The secondary port should be inserted under control with direct vision through the laparoscope.
- Once the secondary ports have been inserted, a maintenance operating pressure of 15 mmHg should be implemented.

SECTION III

OSCE PRACTICE CIRCUITS

CHAPTER 10
PRACTICE
CIRCUIT 1

- Duration – 2 hours 48 minutes.
- Structure – 14 stations × 12 minutes, which includes 2 minutes of initial reading time
- Additional information – At the start of each station, you will have 2 minutes to read the instructions for the task and any additional material.
- In addition to the questions, the mark sheets and revision notes are provided.

MODULE 1: TEACHING

Candidate instructions

This station is with a simulated trainee and will assess the following domains:

- Communication with colleagues
- Information gathering
- Applied clinical knowledge
- Patient safety

A junior trainee has come to the department and would like to know more about the third stage of labour.

You have 10 minutes to explain the third stage of labour including:

1. The components of active and passive management.
2. How to diagnose a prolonged third stage of labour.
3. The techniques and medications that are used in active management of third stage.

Simulated trainee instructions

You are a first-year specialist trainee in O&G beginning your placement on the labour ward department. You know that the third stage of labour is the delivery of the placenta but do not know how long is left before a diagnosis of prolonged third stage is made. You are unsure about what constitutes active and passive management of the third stage. You have heard about gentle cord traction but do not know how to perform it. You remember seeing someone given syntometrine during the third stage when you were on placement.

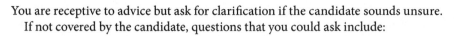

You are receptive to advice but ask for clarification if the candidate sounds unsure. If not covered by the candidate, questions that you could ask include:

- What is the difference between active and passive management of third stage?
- How do you perform gentle cord traction?
- What drugs are used in active third stage?
- Can syntometrine be used for active third stage?

Marking

Communication with colleagues

- Appropriate introduction.
- There should be a clear structure to the delivery of the teaching.
- Encourages learning, discussion and questions with appropriate verbal and non-verbal communication.

Information gathering

- Checks the existing knowledge of the candidate.
- Confirms understanding at appropriate intervals during teaching.

Applied clinical knowledge

- Understands the correct definitions of the third stage of labour and knows what is defined as prolonged third stage.
- Correctly identifies which elements belong to the active and passive third stage of management packages.
- Gives appropriate feedback and develops a learning plan using knowledge of the curriculum and assessment tools.

Safety

- The candidate teaches the importance of counter traction during controlled cord traction of the umbilical cord.
- The candidate should advise that syntometrine should not be given to women suffering from hypertensive disorders due to the risk of further increasing the blood pressure.

Examiner notes

- 'The third stage of labour is the time from the birth of the baby to the expulsion of the placenta and membranes'. (NICE intrapartum guideline)
- Diagnosis of a prolonged third stage of labour is made if expulsion of the placenta and membranes does not occur within 30 minutes of the birth with active management or within 60 minutes of the birth with physiological management.
- Active management of the third stage involves the following components:
  - Use of uterotonic drugs such as 10 IU of oxytocin by intramuscular injection immediately after the birth of the baby.
  - Delayed cord clamping and cutting.

- After signs of separation of the placenta (cord lengthening, gush of blood, uterus becomes smaller and firmer) controlled cord traction is applied (by one hand provides traction and another supports the uterus with suprapubic pressure).
- Physiological management of the third stage involves the following components:
  - Uterotonic drugs are not used routinely.
  - The cord is not clamped until pulsations have stopped.
  - The placenta is delivered by maternal effort.
- For delayed cord clamping, do not clamp the cord earlier than 1 minute from the birth of the baby unless there is concern about the integrity of the cord or the baby has a heart rate below 60 beats/minute that is not getting faster.
- For active management, oxytocin alone is preferred as it is associated with fewer side effects than oxytocin plus ergometrine.

Further reading: NICE intrapartum guideline

MODULE 2: CORE SURGICAL SKILLS

Candidate instructions

This station is a structured viva and will assess your knowledge of instruments used in operative vaginal delivery. It will assess the following domains:

- Communication with colleagues
- Applied clinical knowledge
- Patient safety

The examiner has different pairs of obstetric forceps and will ask you questions regarding forceps delivery. You will be assessed on your ability in answering the questions and the amount of prompting that you require.

Examiner instructions

This is a structured viva of practical skills. The candidate has 12 minutes to answer questions related to operative vaginal delivery using obstetric forceps. You should ask the candidate the questions provided in sequence. The candidate will be provided with the obstetric forceps, a pelvis model and a foetal doll at the beginning of the station. If required, you can prompt the candidate; however, this should be reflected in their overall assessment.

You should be provided the following equipment:

- Kielland's forceps;
- Neville Barnes forceps;
- Pelvic model;
- Foetal doll.

Questions to be asked:

1. Give the candidate the Kielland's forceps (Figure 10.1). Ask the candidate to identify the instrument and to name the key features that facilitate their use (rotational mid-cavity forceps delivery).
2. Give the candidate the Neville Barnes obstetric forceps (Figure 10.2). Ask the candidate to identify the instrument and to give the indications for its use.
3. As a skilled trained operator or obstetric forceps, what are the clinical prerequisites for their safe use.
4. Give the candidate the Neville Barnes obstetric forceps and hold the pelvic model with the foetal doll in a DOA position at +1 station. Ask them to demonstrate a forceps delivery.

Marking

Communication with colleagues

- Clear explanations regarding different forceps.
- Explains concepts well.
- Describes the procedure of forceps delivery in a stepwise sequential manner.

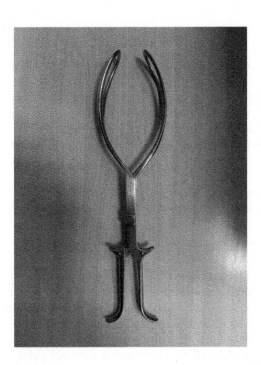

Figure 10.1 Kielland's forceps.

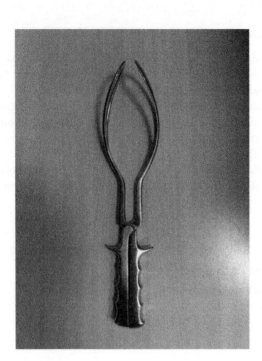

Figure 10.2 Neville Barnes forceps.

Applied clinical knowledge

- Clear understanding of the indications for the use of Kielland's forceps and Neville Barnes forceps.
- Understands the pre-requisites for operative vaginal delivery.
- Candidate shows good clinical knowledge of when forceps delivery is unsuitable or contraindicated.
- Demonstrates familiarity with the conduct of forceps delivery.

Safety

- Understands when forceps should be safely used.
- Demonstrates safe skills when applying forceps and in completing forceps delivery.

Examiner notes

1. *Give the candidate the Kielland's forceps.*
   a. Ask the candidate to identify this instrument and to name the key features that facilitate their use (rotational mid-cavity forceps delivery).
      - Kielland's rotational forceps
      - Rotational delivery of foetuses in an OP or OT position.
      - Sliding lock, cephalic curve and a minimal pelvic curve. The sliding lock allows for correction of asyncliticism and the minimal pelvic curve allows for rotation in the mid-cavity of the pelvis.

2. *Give the candidate the Neville Barnes obstetric forceps.*
   a. Ask the candidate to identify the instrument and give the indications for its use.
      - Non-rotational Neville Barnes forceps.
      - Indications may be divided into foetal and maternal.
      - Foetal indications include: presumed foetal compromise.
      - Maternal indications include: maternal exhaustion, maternal medical conditions restricting second stage of labour or where maternal pushing is discouraged (e.g. maternal cardiac conditions, severe maternal hypertension, spinal cord injury), delay in the second stage of labour.
3. *Ask the candidate, 'As a skilled trained operator or obstetric forceps, what are the clinical pre-requisites for their safe use?'*
   - Head fully engaged with less than or equal to 1/5 palpable per abdomen
   - Full dilatation of the cervix
   - Ruptured membranes
   - An empty maternal urinary bladder
   - Vertex presentation
   - Exact position of vertex known in ROA, LOA, DOA positions
   - Head at or below ischial spines
   - Adequate analgesia (regional anaesthetic or pudendal nerve block)
   - Maternal consent obtained
   - Adequate maternal uterine contractions
4. *Give the candidate the Neville Barnes obstetric forceps and hold the pelvic model with the foetal doll in a DOA position at +1 station. Ask them to demonstrate a forceps delivery*
   - Ensure neonatal doctor in attendance.
   - Position patient in lithotomy position.
   - Check the forceps are a true pair by locking outside of vagina.
   - Apply lubricant to forceps.
   - Empty the urinary bladder.
   - Last vaginal examination to be sure of the foetal position.
   - Apply forceps in an atraumatic manner using a pencil grip in between contractions with a gentle and wide sweep in line with the inguinal ligament. The maternal left blade should be applied first, followed by the maternal right blade. Ensure protection of the maternal vaginal tissues.
   - Ensure blades easily lock. If not, then remove blades and re-apply.
   - In between contractions, relax locking of blades.
   - Check that the sagittal suture is in the midline.
   - Gentle traction at the peak of each uterine contraction with coaching of maternal effort.
   - Right mediolateral episiotomy when delivery imminent on crowning.
   - Traction vector should be in the J-shaped curve of the maternal pelvis, with a horizontal vector at crowning.
   - Coaching of mother to reduce maternal efforts and protection of the perineum.
   - Complete delivery of the head, untangling any cord, if appropriate.

- Deliver shoulders after restitution.
- Deliver the placenta with active third stage management.
- Careful examination of the perineum and vagina.
- Repair perineum.
- Debrief mother.
- Documentation.

Revision notes

You will be expected to perform this station well. Before the exam, try and read up the definitions of lie, engagement, station and position so that they are on the tip of your tongue. We expect undergraduate students to know these definitions so it would be unacceptable for a MRCOG candidate to not know them.

Next time that you are doing a forceps delivery, try and complete it in a textbook manner. Really consider what you are saying to the patient when you are counselling them about the forceps delivery and also what you will say during the forceps delivery. This could quite easily be a role-play station where you are expected to counsel a woman who has had delay in the second stage of labour regarding forceps delivery, which is then linked with a structured viva regarding safe forceps delivery.

As with any practical skill, imagine that you are performing the practical skill in real life. This way, it is less likely that you will forget any of the steps due to nervousness.

MODULE 3: POST-OPERATIVE CARE

Candidate instructions

This task is a structured discussion assessing the following domains:

- Information gathering
- Applied clinical knowledge
- Patient safety
- Communication with patients

You are the ST5 on call for gynaecology at St Elsewhere hospital. You have been called to A&E Department at 8 pm to see a 42-year-old woman who you performed a routine abdominal hysterectomy 2 weeks ago. She is complaining of loss of urinary control and a constant feeling of vaginal wetness necessitating the wearing of sanitary protection.

You have 10 minutes to answer a series of questions from the examiner regarding the management of this woman.

Examiner instructions

This is a structured viva. You should ask the candidate the questions on your mark sheet. You can prompt the candidate if necessary, but this requirement should be reflected in the global marks awarded.

Questions to be asked:

1. What diagnoses do you suspect?
2. What would your next steps be to confirm or refute the diagnosis?
3. A small vesico-vaginal is confirmed on micturating cystogram. The IVU is normal. What would your next steps be in the management of this patient?
4. Now the vesico-vaginal fistula diagnosis is confirmed, you go to speak to the patient. What would you tell the patient?
5. Why can a vesico-vaginal fistula occur?
6. What would you do after care is taken over by the urologists?

Marking

Communication with colleagues

- The candidate should involve the consultant immediately
- The management plan should involve colleagues from other specialities, as appropriate

Information gathering

- The candidate arranges appropriate examination and investigations for a vesico-vaginal fistula.

Applied clinical knowledge

- An appropriate differential diagnosis list should be formulated.
- The candidate should demonstrate knowledge of causes of fistula formation – bladder close to vagina anatomically; a misplaced suture may have incorporated the bladder into the vagina, avascular necrosis as a result of infection/haematoma.

Patient safety

- The candidate should recognise the limitations of their clinical abilities and call senior colleagues appropriately.
- The candidate should demonstrate an understanding of the role of clinical governance in relation to post-operative complications.

Examiner notes

1. What diagnoses do you suspect?
   a. Urinary tract-vaginal fistula (vesico-vaginal, uretero-vaginal).
   b. Urinary tract infection
   c. Pelvic haematoma/abscess (serious discharge)
2. What would be your next steps to confirm or refute the diagnosis?
   a. Take a history
   b. Pelvic examination
   c. MSU
   d. HVS

e. Methylene blue instillation to bladder, visualisation ± swab in vagina
  f. Admit the patient for further imaging
  g. Pelvic ultrasound scan
  h. Micturating cystogram
  i. IVU
3. A small vesico-vaginal fistula is confirmed on micturating cystogram. The intravenous urogram is normal. What would your next steps be in the management of this patient?
  a. Inform consultant
  b. Contact urologists (or urogynaecologist with suitable experience)
  c. Speak to patient
4. Now the vesico-vaginal fistula diagnosis is confirmed, you go to speak to the patient. What would you tell the patient?
  a. The patient needs to be informed as there is a duty of candour to the patient.
  b. Apologise to the patient.
  c. Infrequent but recognised complication. Explain why it has occurred and that care will taken over by specialist.
5. Why can a vesico-vaginal fistula occur?
  a. The bladder is close to vagina anatomically and a misplaced suture may have incorporated the bladder into the vagina.
  b. Avascular necrosis as a result of infection/haematoma.
6. What would you do after the care is taken over by the urologists?
  a. Follow-up the patient – review regularly as an inpatient, see in gynaecology outpatients (do not hide).
  b. Clinical governance – acknowledge unexpected complication

This question not only assesses your clinical experience/knowledge but also (and more importantly) your communication skills.

With any serious complication, you should inform your consultant immediately. Experience is particularly important in these situations. Older, more experienced consultants will often be approached by their more junior consultant colleagues in infrequent or unusual situations for advice, i.e. 'expert' opinion where 'evidence' is lacking, so you should use the hierarchy also.

Most surgeons will take complications directly related to surgery personally. Despite this, you should not 'hide' but keep a high profile and make yourself readily available to the patient and her family. You must give an honest appraisal of the complication (reasons, prognosis) and apologise/empathise.

Try not to contradict what other specialities (in this case urology) may say, but it is reasonable to outline the likely options (if you know them; if not, do not guess!).

MODULE 4: ANTENATAL CARE

Candidate instructions

This station is a role-play station and will assess your abilities to communicate the risks and benefits of vaginal birth after C/S to a simulated patient. You will be assessed using the following domains:

- Patient safety
- Communication with patients and their relatives
- Information gathering
- Applied clinical knowledge

You will see Jane Derbyshire, a 32-year-old woman who has previously had one child – a daughter who is now 3 years old. Her daughter was delivered by C/S at a nearby hospital, and there are no details regarding the delivery. You are told that the Mrs. Derbyshire's daughter was normally grown and that her ultrasound scans so far in this pregnancy are normal.

She is now 32 weeks in to her second pregnancy and wants clarification regarding how she will deliver this baby. You will have 10 minutes to take an obstetric history, discuss the benefits and risks of vaginal birth after C/S and to organise a plan of delivery for Mrs. Derbyshire.

Simulated patient instructions

You are Jane Derbyshire, a 32-year-old marketing manager who is now 32 weeks into your second pregnancy. You have a 3-year-old daughter who was born at another hospital. You went through a long labour for your daughter at 39 weeks gestation when you laboured spontaneously, which eventually ended with an abandoned forceps delivery and emergency caesarean section for which you had to stay in hospital for 3 days for recovery. After discharge, you had no further problems but can remember that you felt a lot of discomfort for the first 2 weeks after your C/S. At birth, you were told that you could attempt another vaginal delivery and that your daughter was a normally grown baby for you.

You are anxious about attempting another vaginal delivery. A friend of yours attempted a vaginal birth after having a C/S and eventually had a second C/S as an emergency.

Your initial wish is to opt for an elective C/S. However, once counselled, you are open to the suggestion of attempting a normal vaginal birth if you should labour spontaneously but would not consider an induction of labour. Your main drivers are the health of yourself and your second baby and your desire to be able to look after your 3-year-old Daisy after your delivery.

You are otherwise fit and well, do not take any regular medications, have no allergies. Apart from the C/S, you have never had any other operations. You are a non-smoker and have not drank any alcohol during your pregnancy.

If not covered by the candidate, questions that you could ask include:

- What is the likelihood of me achieving a normal vaginal birth?
- What are the risks of trying to have a normal delivery after having a C/S previously?
- What are the benefits of trying to have a normal delivery after having a C/S previously?
- Where will I deliver?
- What kind of monitoring will I have?

Marking

Patient safety

- Knowledgeable regarding the risks and benefits of VBAC
- Understands the arrangements that should be made for a woman attempting VBAC (e.g. continuous electronic foetal monitoring, delivery on the labour ward, IV access)
- Arranges appropriate follow-up at around 40 weeks to further discuss induction and to check the on-going management plan. Clearly demonstrates knowledge regarding additional risks with induction

Communication with patients and their relatives

- Demonstrates good communication skills during history taking
- Acknowledges the patient's concerns and anxieties
- Explains the risks and benefits of VBAC in a measured way supplying information in an accurate and balanced manner
- Adopts a mutualistic approach to producing a clear plan for the mode of delivery and how to manage the rest of the pregnancy
- Avoidance of medical jargon throughout
- Ensures the patient understands and is content with the plan for the rest of the pregnancy
- Does not coerce the patient into having a VBAC.

Information gathering

- Demonstrates a clear structure when taking an obstetric history
- Listens to the patient attentively and allows good flow of information
- Assesses the wish of the patient regarding mode of delivery
- Attempts to find out further information regarding the previous C/S at the neighbouring hospital

Applied clinical knowledge

- Understands the risks and benefits of VBAC and elective repeat C/S.
- Demonstrates understanding of additional risks involved with induction of labour in women attempting VBAC

Examiner notes

- In this clinical scenario, the candidate should take a concise obstetric history. This should include POH, PMH, PSH, DH, allergy history, social history
- The thoughts and opinion of the patient regarding mode of delivery should be elucidated and her concerns and anxieties should be acknowledged
- The benefits and risks of VBAC should be discussed
- Benefits
  - 75% of women attempting VBAC will be successful
  - VBAC avoids the risk of planned surgery and their complications
  - Increased chance of uncomplicated pregnancies in the future
  - Lower chance of requiring a blood transfusion
  - Quicker recovery
- Risks
  - Risk of scar rupture is 1 in 200 (0.5%)
  - Risk of perinatal death is extremely low and is comparable to a nulliparous woman in labour
- The candidate should allow time for the patient to consider the information provided and allow opportunities for the patient to ask questions throughout the counselling
- The candidate should counsel the patient regarding the intrapartum management of a woman attempting VBAC.
  - Delivery on a labour ward
  - IV access
  - Availability of neonatal resuscitation and recourse to emergency C/S
  - The use of continuous electronic foetal monitoring
- Once the patient has agreed to have a VBAC, the candidate should make provisions with regard to planning for the rest of the pregnancy. This should include:
  - The patient continuing to see her community midwife at 2 weekly intervals
  - To offer an appointment close to the due date so that induction of labour can be discussed if required with a senior obstetrician or organisation of an elective repeat C/S.
  - Advice regarding what to do at the spontaneous onset of labour.
  - Some form of attempt to gather further information regarding the previous C/S
  - Once the plan has been finalised, the candidate should check understanding with the patient and ensure that the patient is satisfied with the plan for her on-going pregnancy.

Revision notes

You should be able to complete a comprehensive obstetric history fairly quickly in this scenario and realise that you need further information from the patient regarding her previous C/S.

After this, it is important to ask the patient what their initial thoughts are with regard to their preferred mode of delivery. Active listening should be demonstrated by non-verbal communication. Once you have ascertained the wishes of the patient, you should attempt to understand whether a VBAC is an option that the patient would consider. Remember patients may not be open to any other option than an elective repeat C/S.

Your job as a safe candidate is to provide information for the patient to make an informed decision regarding her mode of delivery. Try not to appear to be coercive or overly persuasive in your counselling.

Finally, you should provide the patient with a clear plan for the rest of her pregnancy. Be positive regarding the end of the consultation. There should be no doubt or confusion regarding the on-going plan for the patient. The plan should certainly include some form of communication to investigate the details of the patient's previous C/S and when to meet at antenatal clinic to make further arrangements if spontaneous labour has not occurred.

Further reading: RCOG Green top guideline for VBAC

MODULE 5: MATERNAL MEDICINE

Candidate instructions

This station is with a simulated patient and will assess the following domains:

- Communication with patients
- Information gathering
- Applied clinical knowledge
- Patient safety

You are about to see Shobna Agarawal, a 29-year-old solicitor, who has attended the outpatient department for pre-pregnancy counselling. She was diagnosed with Type 2 diabetes mellitus last year, which is being controlled on the oral hypoglycaemic Metformin.

You have 10 minutes in which you should:

- Take a brief directed history.
- Give appropriate advice regarding management of pregnancy.
- Answer any patient questions.

Simulated patient instructions

You are Shobna Agarawal, a 29-year-old married solicitor. You have never been pregnant before.

You were diagnosed with Type 2 diabetes mellitus last year and this is being controlled with diet and oral medication (Metformin 500 mg TDS). Your last HBA1c result was 68. At the same time, as being diagnosed with Type 2 diabetes mellitus, you were diagnosed with high blood pressure and were started on Lisinopril 20 mg once daily. You have no other medical or surgical history.

You have been having the contraceptive injection (Depo-Provera) for the last 3 years for fertility control. Your periods are infrequent and very light. You last had a cervical smear 7 years ago.

You have a family history of high blood pressure (your mother and father are both on treatment for this). You drink about 4 units of alcohol per week and smoke socially.

You are keen to start a family but are very worried about this, because you have heard that many babies born to diabetic mothers are abnormal. You have also heard that it is better to deliver the baby by a planned elective C/S.

If not discussed by the candidate, the following questions may be helpful:

What are the risks to you and baby if you get pregnant with diabetes?

What can you do to reduce the risks?

Is it better to have a planned elective C/S?

Marking

Communication with patient

- Adequate introduction, good body language and eye contact.
- Able to describe the impact of diabetes on pregnancy while avoiding medical jargon and ensuring patient understanding.
- Addresses concerns of patient in an empathetic manner.

Information gathering

- Takes a concise and relevant history.
- Uses open questions and signposting to direct the consultation.

Applied clinical knowledge

- The candidate should demonstrate knowledge of the impact of diabetes on pregnancy and the foetus.
- Gives general pre-pregnancy counselling advice for Type 2 diabetes mellitus as well as specific information for this patient (stopping smoking, offer smear, contraceptive advice, folic acid and changing hypertensive medication).

Safety

- The candidate should show the ability to safely prescribe in pregnancy by advising to stop the ACE inhibitor and start high dose folic acid.
- Part of the management plan should include the assessment of diabetic control and diabetic complications that will influence when it is safe to get pregnant.

Examiner notes

One of the main difficulties in this task is to complete it within the allotted 10 minutes. To do this, the history has to be focused and cannot take up more than 5 minutes; ideally, it should take less than 4 minutes to complete. The use of structured open questions can achieve this and allow more time to counsel the patient.

The importance of diabetic control pre-conceptually and antenatally

- Pre-conceptual care does improve outcomes (and is cost-effective).
- Optimal metabolic control reduces the risk of miscarriage, congenital malformations and reduces the risk of an unhealthy baby (e.g. hypoglycaemia)
- Give an outline of routine management during pregnancy: attendance and joint diabetic clinics with a named obstetrician and physician and standardised protocols for management; tight blood sugar control (diet and possibly need insulin), hospital assessments; advice re hypoglycaemia management to patient and partner; close surveillance of foetal growth and well-being, BP, urine (infection, proteinuria, glycosuria and ketones).

Pre-pregnancy obstetric advice – general

- Folic acid 5 mg/day (at least 3 months pre-conception and until 12 weeks gestation)
- Stop smoking – referral to smoking cessation service
- Reduce/cease alcohol intake
- Review all medications (including complementary) for safety; advise stopping ACE inhibitor and replacing with another antihypertensive
- Check BP
- Check rubella
- Advise cervical smear (not performed within last 3 years)
- FBC (check for anaemia)

Pre-pregnancy obstetric advice – specific to diabetes

- Contraception
  - Stop the Depo-Provera as it may take up to 1 year for fertility to return
  - Use barrier contraception (or POP/COC) for the next 3 months to allow for folate supplementation and establishment of tight diabetic control.
- Check HbA1c levels – ideally pregnancy should be delayed until HbA1c <48 mmol/mol (6.5%).
- Tight blood sugar targets
- Dietary advice – dietician/nurse specialist
- Aware of dangers of:
  - Hypoglycaemia management must be reviewed particularly if switched on to insulin. Early morning hypoglycaemia is more common in early pregnancy
  - Hyperglycaemia and ketoacidosis

Pre-pregnancy obstetric advice – diabetic complications screening

- Nephropathy:
  - U&Es (high creatinine is associated with poorer pregnancy outcomes)
  - Urine for proteinuria estimation and creatinine clearance
- Retinopathy:
  - Refer to ophthalmologist for an eye examination conducted through dilated pupils

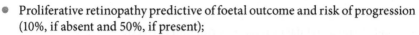

- Proliferative retinopathy predictive of foetal outcome and risk of progression (10%, if absent and 50%, if present);
- Retinopathy requiring treatment should be dealt with prior to pregnancy
- Consider the possibility of macrovascular disease (e.g. IHD, CVA) and formally investigate if it is a possibility.
- Early review when pregnancy confirmed.

Further reading: NICE guideline for diabetes in pregnancy

MODULE 6: MANAGEMENT OF LABOUR

Candidate instructions

This station is a structured VIVA and will assess your abilities to answer questions surrounding the management of labour. You will be assessed using the following domains:

- Patient safety
- Communication with colleagues
- Information gathering
- Applied clinical knowledge

You are the registrar on-call on labour ward. You have been asked to assess a multiparous woman who is failing to make progress in the first stage of labour. The patient is a 35-year-old woman who is in her second pregnancy.

You will have 10 minutes to answer questions that are asked by the examiner. You will be assessed according to your ability in answering the questions and the amount of prompting that you require.

Marking

Patient safety

- Interprets the partogram correctly
- Understands the information required to formulate an on-going plan for labour
- Formulates a safe plan of care for the rest of labour
- Demonstrates understanding of the potential risks of augmentation of labour in a multiparous woman – uterine rupture
- Reacts to sepsis in labour and implements the 'sepsis care pathway'

Communication with colleagues

- Clear explanation of why delay of labour is seen in the partogram provided
- Provides list of information required in a methodical manner
- Clear explanation of concerns regarding uterine rupture, prolonged rupture of membranes and sepsis
- Methodical approach and explanation of on-going plan for the rest of labour

Information gathering

- Able to interpret data from the partogram correctly
- Clear understanding of important factors to take into account when providing list of further information required
- Provides a comprehensive list of examination findings to look for in a woman with suspected chorioamnionitis

Applied clinical knowledge

- Demonstrates knowledge of the NICE intrapartum care guideline and applies this knowledge in the interpretation of the partogram
- Demonstrates knowledge of the seriousness of intrapartum sepsis and the sepsis pathway.

Examiner notes

Ask the questions below to the candidate in the sequence provided.

1. Give the partogram (Figure 10.3) provided to the candidate. Ask the candidate, 'What is this and what does it show?'
   - Labour partogram
   - Patient details
   - Timing of vaginal examinations with dilatation, position, station
   - Contractions
   - Maternal observations
   - Foetal heart rate
   - Evidence of delay in first stage of labour due to inadequate contractions
2. Ask the candidate, 'What additional clinical information would you ask for about this woman?'
   - Antenatal details:
     - Maternal age and BMI/stature
     - Gestation
     - Parity
     - Details regarding previous normal vaginal delivery
     - Any evidence of macrosomia in the antenatal period from symphysio-fundal height measurements or growth scans
   - Intrapartum details
     - Further details regarding induction of labour – what was the indication and how it was performed
     - Progress of labour to date – timing of examinations and their findings
     - The nature and frequency of the contractions
     - CTG findings
     - Analgesia provided
3. Ask the candidate, 'What clinical examination would you perform?'
   - Assess hydration status of patient
   - Abdominal examination to assess for foetal size, presentation and engagement of the foetus

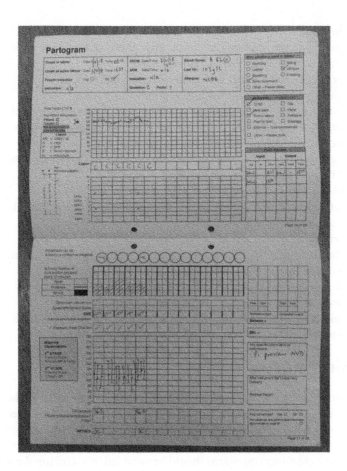

Figure 10.3 Partogram.

- Vaginal examination to assess for signs of cephalopelvic disproportion – moulding and caput and to rule out face or brow presentation
4. Tell the candidate, 'There is evidence of delay in the first stage of labour. What course of action would you take now?'
   - Commence IV rehydration
   - If there are no signs of cephalopelvic disproportion to augment labour with oxytocin infusion
   - The delay in labour is likely due to inadequate contractions
   - The candidate should provide justification for their decision for augmentation and also declare their concerns regarding uterine rupture in view of parity
   - Review in 2 hours to repeat examination of the cervix to assess for effect of oxytocin infusion on contractions and to ascertain whether there had been any progress in labour
   - Continue with continuous electronic foetal monitoring
   - Full explanation of the plan to the woman

5. Tell the candidate, 'When you return to this patient 2 hours later, the CTG is normal but the midwife tells you that there is maternal pyrexia with a temperature of 38.2°C. What do you do now?'
   - Carry out a full clinical assessment. This should include:
   - Assessment of the maternal observations
   - An abdominal examination to assess for continuous uterine tenderness
   - A vaginal examination to assess for progress in labour and to investigate whether the lochia is offensive in smell or appearance.

6. Tell the candidate, 'You suspect that the woman has chorioamnionitis, what would be your next course of action?'
   - Initiate sepsis pathway. This should include:
   - Performing blood cultures and taking blood tests for FBC, U+E, CRP, serum lactate
   - Performing a low vaginal swab
   - Administration of broad spectrum IV antibiotics (e.g. cefuroxime and metronidazole) after ascertainment of allergy history
   - Administering IV fluid therapy
   - Assess foetal well-being
   - Make a judgement as to whether delivery of the foetus will be completed soon or whether intervention by C/S should be undertaken.

Revision notes

This is a common scenario faced by MRCOG Part 3 candidates in their clinical practice. Therefore, you should aim to perform this station very well. A good candidate will be able to interpret the partogram and explain why information that is required and their subsequent management are justified. Furthermore, the answers to the examiners questions should be provided in a structured manner with evidence that you can think about clinical scenarios in a methodical way.

A good candidate should also be able to express their concerns and thoughts regarding uterine rupture and intrapartum sepsis in this clinical context and ensure that patient safety is kept at top priority.

MODULE 7: MANAGEMENT OF DELIVERY

Candidate instructions

This station is a structured discussion and will assess the following domains:

- Communication with colleagues
- Applied clinical knowledge
- Patient safety

You are the ST5 on labour ward and have been called to review Sarah Smith who has been transferred from the midwife-led unit. She is 38 weeks into her second pregnancy and has been fully dilated and pushing for 2 hours. She is using gas and air for analgesia and is becoming increasingly tired and distressed. You perform a vaginal examination that confirms she is fully dilated, with a direct occipitoposterior position, at −1 station, with caput and moulding. A CTG has been started, which is normal.

You have 10 minutes in which to discuss your management for this clinical scenario with the examiner. Examiner will have questions to direct the discussion.

Examiner instructions

Familiarise yourself with the candidate instructions. You should ask the questions in the order given. You may prompt the candidate, but this should be reflected in the marks you give.

1. What is your diagnosis and management plan?
2. You decide to take the patient to theatre for a possible C/S to have full dilatation. What preparations do you make before you begin?
3. What considerations should you have with technique for a C/S performed at full dilatation?

Marking

Communication with colleagues
- An appreciation of the different roles of the multidisciplinary should be demonstrated.
- The WHO checklist should be used to highlight risks to the team.

Applied clinical knowledge
- The candidate should diagnose delay in second stage due to malposition.
- There should be an understanding of the risks of C/S at full dilatation and ways to reduce the risks.
- There should be an appreciation of the techniques needed to deal with a second stage C/S.

Safety
- The candidate should know their limitations and the need to inform the consultant.
- Consent should be taken and the CTG should be checked to determine the category of the C/S.
- The WHO checklist should be performed and used as an opportunity to inform the team of a potentially difficult birth.
- A repeat vaginal examination in theatre is important as things can rapidly change in the second stage.

Examiner notes

Example answers:

1. **What is your diagnosis and management plan?**

   This scenario describes a delay in second stage of labour. The obstructed labour is most likely due to cephalopelvic disproportion caused by the occipitoposterior position. Given the examination findings, the parity and how long the woman has been pushing for, then the decision to take the patient to theatre for a C/S should be made. If the patient does not want a C/S, the consultant should be informed and pain relief offered.

2. **You decide to take the patient to theatre for a possible C/S at full dilatation. What step do you take before you begin?**

   Before beginning the procedure, the following preparations should be made:

   - The consultant on-call should be notified and the most senior obstetrician available should be present in case of a difficult delivery or repair of uterine extensions is necessary.
   - The patient should have IV access with a large bore cannula and, at least, have a valid group and save.
   - On the consent form, as well as the usual risks, there should be an increase in emphasis of major haemorrhage, which is a risk factor in second stage deliveries.
   - During the WHO checklist, the staff should be aware that it is a full dilatation C/S along with the urgency. It should be clear that there is an increased risk of haemorrhage and a potentially difficult birth.
   - A vaginal examination should be performed, as findings can quickly change.
   - The CTG should be checked to help guide the category of the C/S.
   - The neonatal team should be made aware and should be present in theatre for the birth.
   - The anaesthetist should give adequate anaesthesia and should be prepared to give uterine relaxants. The anaesthetist should also be told not only to give a bolus of oxytocin but also provide an oxytocin infusion as soon as the baby is born.
   - Intravenous antibiotics should be given prior to skin incision to reduce the chances of infection.
   - Depending on local policy, an experienced obstetrician or midwife should be available to dis-impact the head or a foetal pillow may be used.

3. **What considerations should you have with technique for a C/S performed at full dilatation?**

   The following should be considered while performing necessary section for allocation:

   - There is an increased risk of extensions to the uterine incision. The bladder should be well reflected both centrally and laterally.
   - The incision on the lower segment should be higher than usual to ensure that you are clear of the cervix and vagina.
   - As the lower segment is likely to be thin and the amniotic membranes are ruptured, care must be taken not to cut the baby. A small incision should be made and the uterus entered using finger rather than a knife.

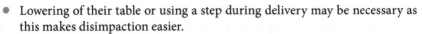

- Lowering of their table or using a step during delivery may be necessary as this makes disimpaction easier.
- During disimpaction your hand should be below the foetal head at the occiput. Disimpaction should only be attempted once the head has been flexed. Traction should be applied towards the mother's head and only when the head is disimpacted, delivery should be attempted.
- If there is difficulty with disimpaction, a second experienced assistant can be requested to flex and push the baby vaginally or by using a foetal pillow.
- If the above techniques have not worked, a reverse breech manoeuvre can be attempted.

MODULE 8: POSTPARTUM COUNSELLING

Candidate instructions

This station is a role-play station and will assess your abilities to counsel the husband of Mrs. Sandra Wu who delivered 2 days ago. Mrs. Wu had prolonged rupture of membranes at 38 weeks gestation for a total of 46 hours. She then underwent syntocinon augmentation. Unfortunately, at 3 cm cervical dilatation, there were signs of foetal distress with large variable deceleration and reduced baseline variability and baseline tachycardia. The decision was made to deliver her by category I emergency CS. The liquor was found to be offensive and the baby was admitted to the neonatal unit and required intubation and ventilation. The neonatologists believe that the baby is septic. Shortly after delivery, Mrs. Wu had a maternal tachycardia of 132 bpm and a temperature of 38.6°C. She is currently being nursed in the HDU and receiving IV antibiotics.

The midwife looking after Mrs. Wu has asked you to speak to her husband who has a few questions surrounding her care.

You will be assessed using the following domains:

- Patient safety
- Communication with patients and their relatives
- Information gathering
- Applied clinical knowledge

You will have 10 minutes to address Mr. Wu's concerns.

Simulated patient instructions

You are Alan Wu, a 33-year-old solicitor. You and your wife attended the hospital a few days ago when Sandra's waters broke. You were surprised at the time that you were asked to go home after that visit to return the next day for induction if labour had not occurred spontaneously. Although you were surprised, you listened to the advice of the midwife that saw you and waited for contractions to occur at home.

When no contractions occurred, you brought Sandra back to the hospital as agreed after 24 hours. You were expecting for labour to be induced and for your baby to be delivered. However, as the hospital was busy, induction was delayed for a further 24 hours.

You are very angry that Sandra was left for such a long time after her waters broke. You believe the reason that she is unwell with infection is because she was left pregnant for such a long period of time. You also think that the reason why your baby is on the neonatal unit with sepsis is because of the same reason. You want to find out what happened and what should have happened when Sandra was admitted after breaking her waters. If the candidate does not deal with your concerns, you wish to make a complaint.

If not covered by the candidate, questions that you could ask include:

- What is the normal management of a woman that has broken their waters who has no contractions?
- Why was she left for such a long time after her waters broke for her to be induced?
- Would the outcomes be the same for mother and baby if you had induced her earlier?
- What will happen now to my wife and my baby?
- Will be there some form of investigation as to whether the poor outcomes could be avoided?

Marking

Patient safety

- Conveys the importance of treating the puerperal sepsis promptly with broad spectrum antibiotics.
- Demonstrates knowledge of when women with PROM should be induced.
- Maintains that the patient's safety during sepsis is currently the primary concern for the obstetric team.

Communication with patients and their relatives

- Acknowledges the patient's anger and frustration
- Apologises for the situation that the patient and her partner find themselves in
- Displays empathy and attentive listening skills
- Allows the patient's partner to vent their feelings without interruption
- Explains that according to guidance that there has been no mismanagement, although this does not mean sepsis cannot occur
- Explains that the primary objective for the obstetric team is to ensure maternal well-being now that there is a puerperal sepsis, likely secondary to chorioamnionitis
- Open and honest manner when addressing the complaint

Information gathering

- Gathers information regarding the concerns and queries from the patient's partner

Applied clinical knowledge

- Demonstrates knowledge of management of pre-labour rupture of membranes at term.
- Understands the need to treat infection promptly and that the patient should stay on HDU for further on-going care with IV antibiotics and full sepsis pathway.

Examiner notes

- In this clinical scenario, the candidate will need to be able to manage a consultation with an angry relative.
- The candidate should allow the patient's partner vent their frustrations, views and opinions without interruption.
- Attentive listening skills should be displayed by the candidate.
- An apology should be made to the partner for what has happened to them and the situation that they find themselves in.
- Once the candidate has dealt with the initial anger, accurate answers regarding the management of PROM should be discussed and how, even in situations where appropriate guidance has been followed, sepsis may still ensue for the mother and the baby.
- The candidate could suggest that the most important objective is now to ensure maternal well-being and to continue with sepsis pathway management.
- Clear explanation of the plan for on-going postnatal care for Mrs. Wu.
- Offer to keep the patient and her partner abreast of developments in the neonatal unit.
- Explain that an incident form will be completed and in clinical situations where there are poor neonatal and maternal outcomes, there will be collection of statements from members of staff that have been involved with clinical care with a subsequent investigation to identify any deficiencies in the delivery of care.
- Offers appropriate advice to Patient and Advice Liaison Services if they wish to make a complaint.

Revision notes

In stations like these, a short introduction of you to the angry patient or relative followed by ample opportunity for them to unload their anger and frustration is the best approach to take. What you must not do is interrupt them as they are venting their anger to you. It is also very easy to feel defensive in these situations but try and avoid this at all costs as it will likely make the angry individual more frustrated. Instead just listen, look sincere and repeat and paraphrase what they have said so that they are aware that you are listening to them. When the role-player has finished venting (which they always will if left long enough), make a sincere apology that they find themselves in their predicament and try and show that you are on their side and want to help them –this can be achieved, by saying something simple like:

> I can see that you are very angry. I am sorry that this has happened to you and I will try my best to try and help you. May I ask you a few questions about what has caused your frustration?.......

When the patient or relative is wrong in their judgement and their anger is not well founded, like in this scenario, it is important not to appear to seem patronising. Instead explain that even though guidelines are followed, occasionally poor outcomes can occur.

Lastly, try and ensure that you explain the risk management procedures that are in place to ensure that poor clinical outcomes have not resulted from substandard clinical care and that the process is an open and honest one. Firstly, an incident form would be logged, followed by review by the risk management team. If required, statements would be collated and an investigation would be conducted to identify whether there were any deficiencies in the care delivered. Offer the avenues by which the patient or relative may complain. This places you on the side of the angry patient or relative and defuses a potential argument or disagreement.

MODULE 9: GENERAL GYNAECOLOGY

Candidate instructions

This station is with a simulated patient and will assess the following domains:

- Communication with patients and families
- Information gathering
- Applied clinical knowledge
- Patient safety

The patient has been referred to the gynaecological clinic by her GP.

Read the referral letter below and obtain a relevant history from the patient. The examiner will then ask you a series of related questions.

> *Dear colleague*
> *Re. Mary Stevens*
> *I would be grateful if you could see this 28-year-old pharmacist who is complaining of dyspareunia since getting married last year. She is keen to start a family and this complaint is preventing her from doing this and is putting a strain on their relationship. I would be very grateful for your opinion and advice on further management.*
> *Yours sincerely*
> *Dr A Prasad*

You have 10 minutes in which you should:

- Take a focused history
- Answer the examiners questions

Simulated patient instructions

You are Mary Stevens, a 28-year-old pharmacist.

You were a virgin when you got married 12 months ago. Sexual intercourse has been a problem ever since you lost your virginity. Specifically, you find penetration very uncomfortable and experienced severe burning in the vagina during sex and are only rarely able to continue. You now find that you are tense prior to sex and this is compounding the situation and affecting your ability to be aroused. You do not enjoy sex as a result and have never had an orgasm. You do not have pain in your abdomen, the pain you experience is very much 'superficial', i.e. vaginal and on the 'outside'.

You have a good relationship with your loving partner, but he is becoming increasingly distant and avoiding intercourse with you because 'he doesn't want to hurt you'. You are upset and worried that he will leave you because of your inability to satisfy him and you want to start trying for a family.

In addition to the painful sex, you have noticed recently that you are experiencing itching and soreness around the outside of the vagina, especially pre-menstrually. You get 'thrush' and urinary tract infections occasionally.

Your periods are fine. You have never tried using tampons but use sanitary towels for menstrual hygiene.

You have no medical problems that you are aware of, in particular, no history of skin diseases. The only surgical history you have is that you did have a 'Bartholin's cyst' drained from your lower vagina as a student 7 years ago. Your smear tests have been normal. You do not smoke or drink alcohol.

Examiner instructions

Familiarise yourself with the candidate's and role-player's instructions. Allow the candidate 5 minutes to take a relevant history and ask the questions on your mark sheet. You may prompt the candidate, but this should be reflected in the marks you give.

Questions you should ask:

1. You examine the patient. On initial inspection, the vulva/vagina appears normal. What differential diagnoses are you considering at present and what further examination findings may support these diagnoses?
2. Your examination and investigations (lower genital tract swabs) are negative. Briefly outline potential management strategies?

Marking

Communication with patient
- Appropriate introduction, listening skills and eye contact.
- Uses open questions and is able to direct the history when appropriate.
- The candidate is able to describe a clear management plan.

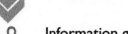

Information gathering

- Uses open questions
- Obtains a directed history that defines the problem and explores potential medical, surgical and psychosocial causes of dyspareunia.

Applied clinical knowledge

- The information given by the history and examiner should be interpreted correctly to give a suitable differential diagnosis.
- The candidate displays knowledge of the treatment for dyspareunia and presents the management options along with their risks and benefits.

Safety

- In the history, the candidate should take steps to screen for physical or sexual abuse.
- There is a risk of a sexually transmitted disease with these symptoms and swabs should be taken to rule this out.

Examiner notes

A directed history should explore the following four key areas with suggestions for a more detailed inquiry, if open questions do not uncover the necessary information:

1. Definition of this dyspareunia and/or concomitant sexual dysfunctions:
   a. Where is the pain located?
   b. When is the onset of pain? (Before entry, vagina, deep or after)
   c. Is it pruritic, burning or aching in quality?
   d. What is the chronological history? If multiple pain sites, which came first?
   e. Has it been a lifelong or acquired?
   f. Are there other sexual dysfunctions such as arousal, lubrication or orgasmic difficulties?
   g. What treatments have been attempted?
2. Exploration of potential gynaecological causes:
   a. Are there vaginal symptoms, including discharge, burning or inching?
   b. Does the patient have a history of STDs, including HSV?
   c. Is there an obstetric delivery history of lacerations, episiotomy or other trauma?
   d. Is there an abdominal or genitourinary (incontinence) surgical or radiation history?
   e. Has the patient had prior gynaecological diagnosis, including endometriosis, fibroids, chronic pelvic pain?
   f. What is the patient's current contraception method and is there any history and of intrauterine device use?
3. Explore potential medical causes:
   a. Is there evidence or history of chronic disease, collagen vascular disorders, autoimmune diseases (diabetes mellitus, thyroid)?
   b. What are the patient's medications: alternative, prescribed, over the counter?

c. Is there alcohol or drug use?

d. Does the patient experience bowel or bladder symptoms?

e. Is there evidence of skin disorders such as eczema psoriasis or other dermatitis?

4. Obtain psychosocial information:

a. What is the patient's view of the problem?

b. Has the problem been present in other relationships?

c. Has the couple been able to discuss the problem? If so, what actions have they tried?

d. Is there any history of sexual or physical abuse?

e. Do life stresses exacerbate the symptoms?

f. Is there evidence of depression or anxiety disorders?

g. What would be considered a satisfactory treatment outcome?

You examine the patient. On initial inspection of the vulva/vagina, it appears normal. What differential diagnoses are you considering at present and what further examination findings may suggest these diagnoses?

Superficial dyspareunia in the absence of all the skin disorders:

- Essential dyspareunia – This is a diagnosis of exclusion.
- Vulvodynia (dysaesthetic [essential] vulvodynia) – NAD or mild erythema, marked tenderness.
- Vulva vestibulitis (subset of vulvodynia) – Erythema, intensity varies; exquisite tenderness on touch of cotton-tipped applicator.
- Vaginismus – Palpable spasm of vaginal musculature; difficulty inserting speculum.
- Atrophic tissue or impaired lubrication – Sparse pubic hair, labial fullness, integrity of vaginal mucosa, vaginal depth, vaginal mucosal friability, fissures; atrophy unlikely in a patient this age without associated symptoms of ovarian failure.
- Infection (acute/chronic infections – Candida, BV, TV, HSV) – discharge, typical lesions, tenderness over urethra/anterior wall of urethritis.
- Vulvovaginal cysts/varicose.
- Bartholins gland – Recurrence, inflammation, scarring from previous surgery (tender/erythema±lesion over Bartholin gland openings).

Your examination and investigations (lower genital tract swabs) are negative. Briefly outline potential management strategies?

- Reassurance (no STI, normal anatomy, other young women have this condition, etc.)
- General measures:
  - Avoid scratching (itch-scratch cycle).
  - Avoid soap, shampoo and bubble bath.
  - Use aqueous cream or emulsifying ointment as a soap substitute.
  - Avoid tightfitting garments.
  - Use cotton underwear and avoid synthetic materials.
  - Avoid use of spermicidal cream/impregnated condoms.

- Use bland, non-irritating moisturiser such as aqueous cream/petroleum jelly.
- After urinating or having a bowel movement, clean the area gently with absorbent cotton or antiseptic wipes. Wipe from front to back (vagina to anus).
- Use tampons rather than sanitary towels.
- Avoid overexertion, heat and excessive sweating.
- Lose weight if appropriate.
- Specific measures:
  - KY Jelly, water-based products, baby oil during intercourse (topical oestrogen cream in old women with vaginitis).
  - Topical local anaesthetic prior to intercourse.
  - Trial of topical steroids to break the 'itch-scratch cycle'.
  - Change diet (avoid allergenic agents such as caffeine beverages, tomatoes, peanuts, dairy).
  - Psychosexual counselling (psychological evaluation, CBT, exploration of negative sexual attitudes, sexual ignorance – discussion of foreplay, arousal phase mechanics, expected sensations, use of mechanical dilators/vibrators).

MODULE 10: SUBFERTILITY

Candidate instructions

This station is a role-play station and will assess your abilities to counsel Mrs. Anne Holmes, a 28-year-old woman who has been diagnosed with subfertility. Mrs. Holmes attended infertility outpatient clinic 3 months ago and baseline infertility investigations were organised for her as she had been trying to conceive with her partner for the past 24 months without success. She has a history of irregular periods for the past 5 years.

Biochemical female fertility investigations, her pelvic ultrasound report and her husband's semen analysis have confirmed polycystic ovarian syndrome as the only cause of her subfertility. Her BMI is 27.

You will be assessed using the following domains:

- Patient safety
- Communication with patients and their relatives
- Information gathering
- Applied clinical knowledge

You will have 10 minutes to address Mrs. Holmes' concerns, explain the diagnosis of polycystic ovarian syndrome and potential treatment options for her.

Simulated patient instructions

You are Anne Holmes, a 28-year-old actress who has been trying desperately for a baby for the past 2 years. It has become the primary focus for your life. You and your husband have been having unprotected sexual intercourse three to four times per week. You have had irregular periods since you stopped taking the combine oral contraceptive pill when you started trying to conceive. You have around five periods per year and each one is very light. Your GP referred you to the infertility clinic after you see her 4 months ago.

When told that you have polycystic ovarian syndrome, you are surprised as you thought that this was only a condition that obese women get. You do not know the scientific background of the condition and want to understand it and ask for explanation from the candidate.

If not covered by the candidate, questions that you could ask include:

- What is polycystic ovarian syndrome?
- How does PCOS affect fertility?
- Can I get pregnant without any treatment?
- I am not obese, so why do I have the condition?
- Why do I need to lose weight?
- How long will it take to get pregnant with the medical treatment?
- What will happen next if I do not get pregnant from the medical treatment?

Marking

Patient safety

- Tries to use non-pharmacological methods to treat PCOS – weight loss
- Admits that they are not sure how to start ovulation-induction agents if they do not know how it is administered
- Or administers it in the correct manner (clomiphene citrate 50 mg OD day 2 to day 6 of the cycle) after progesterone withdrawal bleed

Communication with patients and their relatives

- Acknowledges the patient's hopes for pregnancy
- Explains the concept of PCOS and anovulation in lay language avoiding jargon
- Listens attentively to the patient as they ask questions

Information gathering

- Gathers information regarding what the patient already knows about PCOS
- Gather information about what the patient wishes to know about PCOS

Applied clinical knowledge

- Demonstrates knowledge of PCOS as a clinical condition
- Demonstrates knowledge regarding the management of PCOS

Examiner notes

In this clinical scenario, the candidate should deliver the diagnosis of PCOS and suggest that this is the likely reason why the patient has not conceived

- The candidate should ascertain what the patient knows about PCOS.
- The candidate should explain the concepts of anovulation and PCOS to the patient using simple lay language and avoid jargon.
- Drawing a diagram would be a useful method to explain anovulation and fertilisation.
- The candidate should check the patient's understanding of concepts that have been explained and offer patient information literature.
- The candidate should describe the management options in a structured manner (conservative, medical, surgical-assisted reproductive treatments).
- The options for this patient are weight loss, ovulation induction agents, laparoscopic ovarian drilling and IVF treatment.
- The benefits of weight loss are to increase the chance of regulating ovulation without any risk factors of multiple gestation or side effects of ovulation-induction agents.
- Commonly, clomiphene citrate will be used to induce ovulation. A course of progestogen can be used to induce an endometrial bleed. Clomiphene citrate should then be prescribed to be taken once daily from day 2 of the cycle to day 6. After this, ovulation should be checked for and the couple should then have unprotected sexual intercourse three to four times per week. A total of six ovulatory cycles should be the target. The side effects of ovulation-induction treatment are visual disturbance, jaundice and multiple pregnancy. Approximately 50% of women taking Clomiphene will ovulate and 50% of these women will conceive.
- In women who do not ovulate on Clomiphene, metformin can be added or Letrozole can be used as an alternative. Laparoscopic ovarian drilling is an option where medical ovulation induction is not successful.
- Finally, IVF treatment is an option. The risks of IVF are with oocyte retrieval and ovarian hyperstimulation syndrome.

Revision notes

Examiners will be looking for you to be able to explain difficult concepts well in stations like these. Drawing diagrams to explain concepts is a very useful strategy in the exam. In this station, you could quite easily draw a simple diagram of the uterus, tubes and ovaries and show that if ovulation does not occur fertilisation and pregnancy cannot ensue. Thereafter, try and describe management options in a structured way – starting with the least invasive to the most.

By the end of the consultation, you must try and reach a positive end with a decision regarding ongoing management. Try and also offer some written information for the patient to leave with.

MODULE II: SEXUAL AND REPRODUCTIVE HEALTH

Candidate instructions

This station is with a simulated patient and will assess the following domains:

- Communication with patients
- Information gathering
- Applied clinical knowledge
- Patient safety

You are about to see Mary Emms, a 25-year-old nulliparous psychology student in your gynaecology outpatient clinic who is requesting a termination of an unwanted pregnancy.

You have 10 minutes in which you should:

- Take a brief directed history
- Give appropriate advice regarding her management options
- Answer any patient questions

Simulated patient instructions

You are Mary Emms, a 25-year-old nulliparous psychology student. You are very distressed to find yourself pregnant. You are in a steady relationship with your boyfriend and have been taking combined oral contraceptive for a year, although you do occasionally forget to take one. You are not taking any other medication or supplements. You have no other medical or surgical problems. Your mother has had breast cancer but there is no other medical history in the family. You do not smoke, drink or take drugs.

You are adamant that you do not want to be pregnant but are concerned about the physical (particularly the effect on your future fertility) and psychological effects of termination of pregnancy. You have discussed things with your boyfriend and no one else, and you both want to terminate the pregnancy.

If not covered by the candidate, the following questions could be useful:

- What are the risks of having an abortion?
- Are there better options for a contraceptive than the pill?

Marking

Communication with patient

- Adequate introduction, good body language and eye contact.
- The candidate should take a sensitive, non-judgemental approach
- Addresses concerns of patient in an empathetic manner.

Information gathering

- Takes a relevant gynaecological and sexual health history.
- Uses open questions and signposting to direct the consultation.

Applied clinical knowledge

- The candidate should be able to discuss the different options for TOP and their associated risks.
- Post termination of pregnancy contraception should be discussed to avoid a recurrence. The candidate should demonstrate knowledge of the pros and cons of different forms of contraception.

Safety

- The investigation and/or treatment of PID should be considered.
- There should be a sensitive investigation to how the pregnancy occurred and the decision to have the termination to ensure no coercion.

Examiner notes

In these sorts of counselling/management situations, where there is a finality of the decision (TOP, sterilisation, etc.), it is important to allow patients time to reflect on the information discussed at the consultation. The verbal information should be supported by accurate, impartial printed information.

Regarding the abortion decision, clinicians counselling women requesting abortion should try to identify those who require more support in decision-making thinking be provided in the routine clinical setting (such as those with psychiatric history, poor social support or evidence of coercion). Care pathways for additional support, including access to social services, should be available.

If you have a moral objection to TOP, then professional behaviour dictates that you offer referral to another colleague. You should take an appropriate history to identify medical/surgical risk factors and discuss the potential side effects associated with TOP. You should not give moral or judgemental opinions in your capacity as a clinician. There are other appropriate forums for this.

Do not forget post-TOP contraception and risks of sexually transmitted infections. The consequences of untreated infection can be serious and include pelvic inflammatory disease and subsequent infertility. Therefore, those women undergoing TOP's should be screened and/or treated for PID-related organisms.

An outline for consultation and management of this case includes:

- Sensitive, discrete, non-judgemental approach.
- Accurate, impartial verbal information supported by written advice.
- Convey an emphasis on the duty of confidentiality/discretion of healthcare professionals.
- Explore sensitivity reasons for 'social' termination of pregnancy. Ask if they have been discussed with close friends/family.

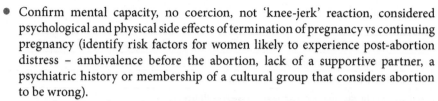

- Confirm mental capacity, no coercion, not 'knee-jerk' reaction, considered psychological and physical side effects of termination of pregnancy vs continuing pregnancy (identify risk factors for women likely to experience post-abortion distress – ambivalence before the abortion, lack of a supportive partner, a psychiatric history or membership of a cultural group that considers abortion to be wrong).
- Discuss risks and sequelae of abortion in order to give valid consent:
  - Haemorrhage in 1 in 1000 abortions at this gestation; uterine perforation 1–4 in 1000; cervical trauma 1 in 100; failed abortion and continuing pregnancy (for surgical TOP 2 in 1000; for medical TOP 1–14 in 1000); post-abortion infection: genital tract infection, including pelvic inflammatory disease.
  - Infections of varying degrees of severity occurs in up to 10% of cases without prophylaxis/bacteriological screening; may be associated with a small increase in the risk of subsequent miscarriage or preterm delivery but reassure no other adverse reproductive outcomes (e.g. infertility); possible increased psychological sequelae (psychiatric illness or self-harm, although contentious).
- Discuss management options:
  - Surgical TOP – suction (GA or conscious sedation).
  - Medical TOP – Mifepristone and misoprostol.
  - Testing and/or treatment for PID.
- Discuss post-TOP contraception:
  - IUCD at surgical TOP (Mirena or copper coil).
  - Depot provera.
  - Implants.
  - Oral daily contraceptives (POP, COC) but as failed probably not the best option.
- The patient should initiate treatment within 2 weeks of presentation.

Further reading: RCOG guideline Best practice in abortion and FSRH guidelines on contraception

MODULE 12: EARLY PREGNANCY

Candidate instructions

This station is a role-play station and will assess your ability to interpret the data presented, your ability to communicate with the patient and discuss management options. You are the gynaecology registrar on-call and have been called to the Early Pregnancy Assessment Unit to see Miss Jade Williams, a 29 year-old-woman who has attended with light per vaginal bleeding. She has just had an ultrasound scan of her pelvis and the report is provided below:

Pelvic ultrasound scan report:

Early Pregnancy Scan: Transabdominal/Transvaginal pelvic ultrasound	
Jade Williams DOB: 25/05/1988	
Source: Early Pregnancy Assessment Unit	
Indication: Threatened miscarriage? Assess viability	
Reported by: Alice Gordon	
Gestation sac: Seen	**Endometrium**: Thickened
Position: Normal	**Uterus**: Normal
Volume: 10 mL	**Free fluid**: No
Yolk sac: Seen	**Right ovary**: Seen, normal
Foetus: Seen	**Left ovary**: Seen, normal
Foetal heart activity: Not seen	
CRL: 9 mm	

Report Summary: There is a singleton pregnancy seen within the endometrial cavity. The sac appears irregular and contains a foetal pole – approx. 7 weeks gestation. NO FETAL HEART BEAT SEEN. Confirmed by Susan Hogan

You will be assessed using the following domains:

- Patient safety
- Communication with patients and their relatives
- Information gathering
- Applied clinical knowledge

You will have 10 minutes to explain to Jade the results of her pelvic ultrasound scan; take a gynaecology history and discuss the management options that are available.

Simulated patient instructions

You are Jade Williams, a 29-year-old account manager who has been trying for a pregnancy with your boyfriend for the past 3 months. You were very excited about becoming pregnant after such a short period of time trying to conceive. This is your first pregnancy. Your last period was 9 weeks ago, and you had been having morning sickness up to around two-and-a-half weeks ago. You experienced some light bleeding in the morning and were referred to your GP to the Early Pregnancy Assessment Unit. Your GP told you that everything was likely to be fine and was very reassuring. When you are told that you have suffered a miscarriage, you are shocked at the news as you were expecting the ultrasound scan to be normal. You react in a quiet manner and are subdued by the news requiring some time to process the information.

You are open to all of the management options and would like to know the pros and cons of each management option. You would prefer to avoid surgery, as you are scared at the prospect of having a general anaesthetic. You wish to go home to consider your options before making a final decision regarding how you would prefer to have your miscarriage managed.

You want to know why the miscarriage has happened and are worried that you may not be able to carry a pregnancy and are not sure how you will communicate the news to your boyfriend who was as excited about the pregnancy as you.

If not covered by the candidate, questions that you could ask include:

- This must be some kind of mistake, are you sure that the ultrasound report is mine?
- Why did this happen to me?
- Will I be able to get pregnant again?
- What if I can't carry a baby?
- What will happen now?
- What are the risks and benefits of conservative/medical and surgical management of miscarriage?
- How am I going to tell my boyfriend what has happened?
- Can I come back later to tell you how I want my management to go ahead?

Marking

Patient safety

- Interprets data from the ultrasound scan report correctly
- Correctly identifies that the report has been verified by two sonographers
- Conveys accurate information regarding the risks and benefits of the different miscarriage management options

Communication with patients and their relatives

- Delivers the bad news regarding miscarriage in a sensitive manner
- Allows time for the patient to process delivered information
- Demonstrates effective communication skills throughout
- Listens attentively to the concerns and worries of the patient
- Takes a full gynaecological history
- Explains the management options in a structured way
- Ends the consultation appropriately

Information gathering

- Interprets the ultrasound report correctly
- Gathers a concise gynaecological history effectively
- Collects the views and opinions of the patient regarding her potential management options

Applied clinical knowledge

- Makes the correct diagnosis of missed miscarriage
- Understands the different management options available to the patient
- Demonstrates understanding of the pros and cons of the differing management options for missed miscarriage

Examiner notes

- The candidate should find out what the patient already knows of the clinical situation
- An appropriate warning shot should be given with the diagnosis of missed miscarriage
- An appropriate amount of time should be allowed for the patient to process the news, with appropriate use of silence
- The candidate should ideally seek permission to continue with the consultation
- A structured concise gynaecological history should be taken from the patient including LMP, gravidity and parity, PC, HPC, smear history, STI history, PMH, PSH, DH, allergies, SH, desire for pregnancy
- The candidate should then offer the management options that are available and discuss the risks and benefits of each:
  - Conservative – Least invasive and most natural. May take time and not be successful, requiring further medical or surgical management. Patient will experience pain and bleeding as the miscarriage completes
  - Medical management – Involves taking vaginal tablet pessaries to make the womb contract. Is less invasive than surgical management. May take some time for the pregnancy to be expelled from the womb. Patient will experience some pain and bleeding as the miscarriage completes
  - Surgical management (Manual Vacuum Aspiration, Figure 10.4) – Allows quick resolution of the miscarriage. More invasive than medical and conservative management options and holds the risk of surgery (pain, bleeding, uterine perforation). Can be done with cervical anaesthetic or general anaesthetic

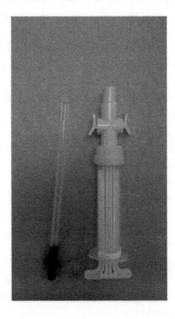

Figure 10.4 Manual vacuum aspirator.

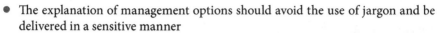

- The explanation of management options should avoid the use of jargon and be delivered in a sensitive manner
- Time should be provided for the patient to digest the information provided
- A patient information leaflet can be provided to aid decision making
- The patient should be reassured that miscarriage is a common occurrence affecting 1 in 4 pregnancies
- It should be explained that most miscarriages are due to genetic abnormalities with the pregnancy rather than there being any maternal cause
- Appropriate reassurance should be provided that the patient will be able to get pregnant again and that the likelihood is that she will go on to carry a baby to full term
- The candidate should accept the suggestion that the patient wishes to go home and think about her options as this also provides some time for conservative management of the miscarriage

Revision notes

One would expect a gynaecological Speciality Trainee of Year 1–2 to be able to perform this station well. A Part 3 MRCOG candidate would be expected to perform this station extremely well. You must effectively analyse the data from the ultrasound report, communicate the bad news of miscarriage in a sensitive way, displaying empathy and allowing time for the patient to take in the bad news.

Thereafter, a simple quick gynaecological history should be obtained, ensuring that all important facets of the patient's history is collected. Explanation of the different management options is key and information should be broken down into digestible chunks.

Miscarriage is just as much a life-changing event as cancer, so the same communication skills are required to deliver this bad news.

Further reading: NICE ectopic and miscarriage guidance CG 157

MODULE 13: ONCOLOGY

Candidate instructions

This station is with a simulated patient and will assess the following domains:

- Information gathering
- Communication with patients
- Applied clinical knowledge
- Patient safety

You have been asked to see Mary Devall, a 58-year-old woman who is presented with intermenstrual bleeding. Her BMI is 35 but has no other medical problems. When she was seen previously, an endometrial biopsy was taken and the results are shown below.

Pathology report

Patient name: Mary Devall

 DOB: 02/02/1960 (Age: 58)

 Clinical details: intermenstrual bleeding

 Specimen: pipelle biopsy

 Gross description: Multiple pieces of tan-red tissue mixed with haemorrhagic material

 Microscopic diagnosis: Endometrioid adenocarcinoma

You have 10 minutes to do the following:

1. Explain the histology findings.
2. Formulate and explain a management plan to the patient.
3. Answer any questions the patient has.

Simulated patient instructions

You are Mary Devall, a 58-year-old pharmacist. You live with your husband David and have two sons who are both at university. You went through the menopause at age 50 but have recently begun to get vaginal bleeding. You have had three episodes of vaginal bleeding; two times it has only been spotting, but on the last occasion, it was like a period. You have also noticed some mild lower abdominal pain at the time of bleeding, but otherwise you have not had any other symptoms. You have always been on the heavy side and have not noticed any weight change. After having an ultrasound scan, you had a biopsy of your womb. You have had no problems since the biopsy.

You are normally fit and well and have an active lifestyle. You have been using hormone replacement therapy since you went through the menopause. You are taking no other medication and have no allergies. You do not smoke and have 2–3 glasses of wine at the weekend. You have no family history of medical problems.

You are very worried about having cancer and are very pessimistic about any diagnosis.

If not discussed by the candidate the following questions may be useful:

- *Do I have cancer?*
- *Am I going to die?*

Marking

Information gathering

- The candidate should take a history relevant to the diagnosis (see below).
- The histology report should be interpreted correctly.

Communication with patients

- Deals with the patient sensitively and offers to meet again with their partner or friend.

- Uses appropriate warning shot(s) before breaking bad news and gives time after to allow the information to sink in.
- Give the patient information in manageable amounts and deals sensitively with and questions.
- The candidate describes the management plan clearly.

Applied clinical knowledge
- The candidate should be able to use the data to formulate an appropriate management plan.
- They should appreciate and convey to the patient that further imaging (MRI) is needed before definitive management plan can be made during a cancer multidisciplinary meeting (MDT).
- They should give a brief description of the cancer MDT.

Patient safety
- The candidate should recognise that endometrial cancer can be oestrogen-sensitive and HRT should be stopped.
- There should be an understanding of the correct referral pathways and treatment targets.

Examiner notes

The most important part of this station is the way you counsel the patient and break the bad news. It is important not to appear rushed and try to be honest. This means not just saying what you do know but also being honest and admitting what you do not know. Do not give inappropriate reassurance or use euphemisms for cancer, e.g. 'little ulcer' when you mean cancer. It is important to listen to the patient and be reactive to any emotional cues. Be prepared to follow the patient's agenda and do not block emotional expression.

A directed history should explore current symptoms, risk factors for development of endometrial cancer (diabetes mellitus, PCOS, hormonal replacement, nulliparity, early menarche, late menopause, hypertension, family history of cancer, smoking and obesity). It should establish risks for surgery such as other medical conditions and previous abdominal surgery as well as social support networks. If the woman was premenopausal, it would be important to determine her fertility desires. Below is an example history framework you can use for a patient with a gynaecological cancer:

History taking
- Oncology
  - How have you been?
  - Any bleeding, weight gain/loss (have you had any changes in your weight), bloating
- Past O&G history
  - Have you had normal smear tests?
  - Have you ever been pregnant?

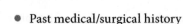
- Past medical/surgical history
  - Do you have any medical problems?
  - Have you had any operations in the past?
- Drug history
  - Are you taking any medications at the moment
  - Do you have any drug allergies
- Family history
  - Do any illnesses/cancers run in the family
- Social history
  - Do you drink or smoke?
  - Who do you live with? Establish support network

Outlook and management for endometrial cancer

Endometrial cancer is the most common gynaecological cancer and should be familiar to all gynaecologists. The overall survival for endometrial cancer is good with 90% surviving 1 year and 80% surviving 5 years. This is because presentation often occurs at an early stage, usually with abnormal uterine bleeding. To stage the cancer, imaging is required usually in the form of an MRI scan. Once the MRI is performed, there will be a discussion of the imaging and histology in the MDT to decide further management. Further management will usually involve a total hysterectomy and bilateral salpingo-oophorectomy with or without lymph node dissection. Where the hysterectomy is performed and whether this is done laparoscopically will depend on the stage, type of cancer and size of the uterus.

MODULE 14: UROGYNAECOLOGY AND THE PELVIC FLOOR

Candidate instructions

This station is a structured VIVA and will assess your abilities to answer questions surrounding pelvic organ prolapse

You will be assessed using the following domains:

- Patient safety
- Communication with colleagues
- Information gathering
- Applied clinical knowledge

You are the gynaecology registrar in the urogynaecology clinic. You will see Mrs Paula Smith, a 62-year-old woman who is complaining of a dragging sensation vaginally. The GP has examined Mrs Smith already and found that she has pelvic organ prolapse. You will be provided data to interpret and then have 10 minutes to answer questions regarding your assessment and management of women with pelvic organ prolapse. You will be assessed according to your ability in answering the questions and the amount of prompting that you require.

Marking

Patient safety
- Understands the need for a comprehensive history to ensure the patient is a safe surgical candidate
- Understands the risks of prolapse surgery

Communication with colleagues
- Provides structured answers to the questions asked
- Communicates the interpreted data in a methodical manner

Information gathering
- Gathers important information from the patient's history to assess for the risk of pelvic organ prolapse
- Understands the important facets of the obstetric history to gather
- Gathers information regarding the examination required in the patient

Applied clinical knowledge
- Demonstrates knowledge of the risk factors for pelvic organ prolapse
- Is able to interpret the POP-Q data and understands the need for POP-Q assessment
- Demonstrates sound knowledge of the risks of pelvic organ prolapse surgery

Examiner notes

Ask the questions below to the candidate in the sequence provided.

1. What information would you like to gather concerning Mrs. Smith?
   - Duration and severity of her symptoms
   - Urinary symptoms
   - Bowel symptoms
   - Sexual symptoms
   - Exacerbating features
   - Menopausal status
   - Any post-menopausal bleeding
   - Use of hormone replacement therapy
   - POH/PMH/PSH/DH/Allergies/SH/FH
2. What in particular would you want to know from her past obstetric history?
   - Parity
   - Modes of delivery – Need for operative vaginal delivery
   - Birth weights
3. What examination would you perform on Mrs. Smith?
   - General examination including:
     - Urinalysis
     - BMI
     - General health

- Post void residual urine volume
- Abdominal examination for the presence of any masses
- Speculum examination with Cusco speculum assessing for vault prolapse and Sims speculum for the assessment of anterior and posterior compartment prolapse
- POP-Q and valsalva test/cough stress test at rest and on reduction of prolapse

4. Can you tell me what the POP-Q assessment is and why it is useful?
   - A method of quantifying prolapse
   - Uses hymen as fixed point of reference – above is a negative number and below is a positive number
   - Compare outcomes of surgical repair
   - Inter examiner reliability and reproducibility
   - Sets standards in publications and presentations
5. Show the candidate the POP-Q provided:

0	0	−5
4	3	8
−3	−3	−6

Can you explain the nature of the POP-Q data here and the diagnosis for Mrs. Smith?

The POP-Q grid shows that Mrs. Smith has a moderate cystocoele

The candidate should know what each box of the POP-Q assessment shows:

Aa −3 normal	Ba −3 normal	C − cervix
GH genital hiatus	PB − perineal body	TVL total vaginal length
AP is −3 normal	BP −3 normal	D posterior fornix

6. What are the management options for Mrs. Smith? If the candidate has not identified a moderate cystocoele, inform him/her of the diagnosis
   - Conservative treatment:
     – Weight loss
     – Pelvic floor exercises
     – Physiotherapy
     – Pessary ring would be advised
     – Combination of above
   - Surgical management
     – Anterior repair
7. Mrs. Smith chooses to have an anterior repair. What are the risks that you would counsel her about?
   - Bleeding
   - Infection
   - Pain
   - Scarring

- Dyspareunia
- Failure of surgery to achieve desired effect
- Recurrence
- Incontinence

Revision notes

You should have a basic understanding of the POP-Q assessment. Even though urogynaecology is a subspeciality of gynaecology, it is reasonable to ask you to interpret data to arrive at the correct diagnosis. This station will mainly assess your ability to communicate with the examiner and provide structured answers. Do not forget the simple treatments for prolapse, as they are just as important as the surgical treatments.

CHAPTER 11
PRACTICE
CIRCUIT 2

- Duration – 2 hours 48 minutes.
- Structure – 14 stations × 12 minutes, which includes 2 minutes of initial reading time
- Additional information: at the start of each station, you will have 2 minutes to read the instructions for the task and any additional material.
- In addition to the questions, the mark sheets and revision notes are provided.

MODULE 1: TEACHING

Candidate instructions

This station is a structured discussion and will assess the following domains:

- Communication with colleagues
- Information gathering
- Applied clinical knowledge
- Patient safety

You have been asked to plan a teaching session for 20 final year undergraduates starting their O&G placement on obstetric abdominal examination. You should base the teaching on the following clinical scenario:

A 30-year-old schoolteacher attends the midwife antenatal clinic at 32 weeks' gestation. There are adequate foetal movements but the midwife is concerned that the uterus feels small for dates. The patient is a smoker and admits to smoking 20 cigarettes per day. Her antenatal care to date has been uneventful.

You have 10 minutes to discuss how you would teach obstetric abdominal examination including:

1. Consideration of setting and teaching style.
2. Details of how to measure the symphysio-fundal height and where to auscultate the foetal heart.

Examiner instructions

The candidate has been asked to plan a teaching session for around 20 undergraduates on abdominal examination. Consideration should be given to the logistics and setting for teaching the students and also the contents. They should demonstrate an understanding of the obstetric abdominal examination and have specifically been asked to give details of how to measure the symphysio-fundal height and where to auscultate the foetal heart. If not covered by the candidate, they can be prompted on these points.

If not covered by the candidate, questions that you could ask include the following:

- Where are you going to do the teaching?
- How will you incorporate the case into the teaching?
- What components of the obstetric abdominal examination will you teach?
- Explain how a symphysio height is measured.

Marking

Communication with colleagues

- There should be a clear structure to the delivery of teaching.
- Chooses appropriate setting avoiding real patients for such a big group but allows practice on models and feedback.

Applied clinical knowledge

- Obstetric examination of the abdomen is a basic skill so the candidate should show familiarity with the steps.
- Develops a learning plan at the end to reinforce teaching.

Safety

- The students should know to take consent before examination and have a chaperone present.
- Is able to describe the correct technique for symphysio-fundal height measurement.
- The candidate should be able to explain where to auscultate the foetal heart.

Examiner notes

Given the large group size teaching in the clinical setting, such as the antenatal department, would be inappropriate. When learning practical skills it is important for the participants to actively take part. This could take the form of an introduction and demonstration from the teacher followed by practice on a model by the student with feedback. An outline of an obstetric abdominal examination is provided below. Models are available for measuring the SFH, and the students could be asked to plot the growth on a customised chart. This could be related back to the clinical case, which would provide an opportunity to teach the reasons behind and management of intrauterine growth restriction. At the end of the teaching, the students should be directed towards opportunities to reinforce their learning such as following a doctor or midwife in antenatal clinic and practicing obstetric examinations.

Obstetric abdominal examination

Wash hands/Introduce yourself/Obtain informed consent for the examination.

General well-being

- Hands: Swelling/pallor/pulse/BP/CRT
- Face: Jaundice/anaemia (conjunctiva)/periorbital oedema
- Leg oedema

Inspection

- Position patient supine
- Expose from the xiphisternum to the pubic symphysis
- Abdomen distended consistent with pregnancy of an appropriate gestation
- Foetal movements
- Surgical scars, e.g. appendicectomy, laparoscopy
- Signs of pregnancy:
  - Line nigra – Dark line from the xiphisternum to the pubic symphysis, due to increased pigmentation
  - Striae gravidarum – Stretch marks

Palpation

Ask for pain before starting

Lie – Relationship between the longitudinal axis of foetus and mother

- Longitudinal (resulting in either cephalic or breech presentation)
- Oblique (unstable, should ideally become either transverse or longitudinal)
- Transverse (resulting in shoulder presentation)

Feel the maternal abdomen to feel which side is the back, i.e. which side of the abdomen feels more full and similar to a smoother structure, i.e. back. This is compared to the other side, where limbs can be felt, including movements.

Presentation – Identify the anatomical part of the foetus that is closest to the pelvic inlet

This could be cephalic, breech or malpresentation, e.g. limb. It is felt by placing thumb and fingers on either side of the presenting part.

Engagement – 'how many 5/5th palpable?'

- Divide the foetal head into fifths ~1 finger width = 1/5th.
- If all of the foetal head is felt in the abdomen, i.e. '5/5th palpable per abdomen'.
- If two finger widths of the foetal head is felt in the abdomen, i.e. '2/5th palpable per abdomen' = engaged.
- If none of the foetal head is felt in the abdomen, i.e. '0/5th palpable per abdomen'.
- The head is engaged when the widest part (the biparietal diameter) has passed through the pelvic brim.

Symphysio-fundal height

- Palpate using ulnar border of left hand moving from sternum downwards.
- Locate the fundus of the uterus (firm feeling).
- Locate upper border of pubic symphysis.
- Place the tape upside down to avoid error.
- Start from the ulnar border of your left hand at the fundus and measure down until you reach the pubic symphysis.
- Measure the distance in cm.
- The distance should correlate with gestational age (±2 cm) but can be measured more accurately on a customised growth chart.

Auscultation

- Once you've identified the lie of the foetus and where the back is, listen over the anterior shoulder of the foetus.
- Use some gel and a sonicaid to listen for 1 minute for the baseline heart rate.

Finish

- Wipe the gel away from both the patient's abdomen and the sonicaid probe.
- Clean the sonicaid probe.
- Wash hands/Thank the patient!/Offer her help to sit back up.
- Discuss findings with the patient ± reassure her.
- Summarise findings.

MODULE 2: SURGICAL SKILLS

Candidate instructions

This station is a structured VIVA and will assess your knowledge of endoscopic surgery. It will assess the following domains:

- Communication with colleagues
- Applied clinical knowledge
- Patient safety

The examiner has different endoscopes used in gynaecological surgery and will ask you questions regarding their use. You will be assessed on your ability in answering the questions and the amount of prompting that you require.

Marking

Communication with colleagues

- Clear explanations regarding the use of different endoscopes and the technique in their use.

- Explains concepts well.
- Describes the procedure of hysteroscopy and cystoscopy well.

Applied clinical knowledge

- Understands the indications for hysteroscopy and cystoscopy.
- Understands the techniques employed and features associated with the different endoscopes.
- Demonstrates familiarity with performing hysteroscopy and cystoscopy.

Safety

- Understands when hysteroscopes and cystoscopies should be used.
- Demonstrates safety when describing the performance of hysteroscopy and cystoscopy.

Examiner instructions

This is a structured VIVA of practical skills. The candidate has 10 minutes to answer questions related to gynaecological endoscopic surgery. You should ask the candidate the questions provided in sequence. The candidate will be provided with a rigid 30° 5 mm diagnostic hysteroscope and a rigid cystoscope. If required, you can prompt the candidate; however, this should be reflected in their overall assessment.

You should be provided the following equipment:

- A rigid 5 mm diagnostic hysteroscope
- A rigid cystoscope

Structured VIVA questions

1. *Give the candidate the diagnostic hysteroscope* (Figure 11.1)
   a. Ask the candidate to identify this instrument and to name the key features that facilitate their use.
      - Diagnostic hysteroscope

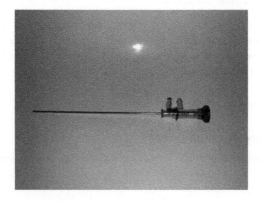

Figure 11.1 Diagnostic hysteroscope.

- Rigid telescope
- Proximal eye piece
- 30° distal lens
- Port for light source
- Inflow port

b. Ask the candidate to give the indications of its use.
- Abnormal uterine bleeding
- Post-menopausal bleeding
- Infertility
- Recurrent pregnancy loss
- Abnormal glandular cervical smears

c. Ask the candidate to describe how a hysteroscopy should be performed.
- Lithotomy position
- Clean and drape the patient
- Prepare the hysteroscope by attaching the light lead to illuminator and saline into the inflow port. Attach the camera and check if the image is in focus and of adequate quality
- Fix cervix with vulsullum
- Commence flow of saline
- Introduce distal lens into cervical canal
- Advance hysteroscope under direct vision using the flowing saline to distend the cervical canal
- Ensure entry into the uterine cavity and remove vulsullum
- Allow for the image to clear
- Perform a 360° view of the uterine cavity by adjusting the light lead to angle the lens towards visual target. Ensure that the both tubal ostia, fundus, anterior, posterior, lateral walls, isthmus have been inspected
- Capture images of important structures
- Remove hysteroscope

2. *Give the candidate the rigid cystoscope* (Figure 11.2)
   a. Ask the candidate to identify the instrument and describe its key features that facilitate its use.
   - Rigid cystoscope
   - Telescope within an obturator, allowing introduction into the urethral meatus
   - Angle of distal lens – Usually 70° to allow for acute angle views
   - Bridge – Allows locking between the inner telescope and the outer obturator
   - Light source attachment
   - Inflow port
   - Operating channels to allow cannulation of the ureteric orifices

   b. Ask the candidate to give the indications of its use.
   - Urinary symptoms – Frequency, chronic dysuria, haematuria
   - Suspected operative trauma
   - Suspected bladder lesions
   - Staging for malignancy

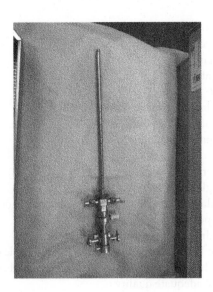

Figure II.2 Rigid cystoscope.

c. Ask the candidate how they would perform a diagnostic cystoscopy.
   — Lithotomy position.
   — Clean and drape.
   — Prepare cystoscope by attaching the light lead to illuminator and saline into the inflow port. Attach the camera and check if the image is in focus and is of adequate quality.
   — Remove the telescope from the obturator.
   — Apply lubrication to obturator and gently insert into bladder for emptying.
   — Once bladder empty, insert telescope into obturator and lock bridge.
   — Start distension with saline under direct vision.
   — Systematic inspection of the bladder – Bladder neck, trigone, ureteric orifices interureteric ridge, bladder floor, fundus and lateral walls. Adjusting the light lead rather than moving the telescope excessively obtains views of these structures.
   — Capture images of important structures.
   — Take note of volume of distension.

Revision notes

Most registrars that are sitting the MRCOG Part 3 will be able to perform well in this station. A good candidate will have good knowledge of endoscopes and will be well versed on their features and know why they may be used. Once again, for practical skills, imagine you are in the clinical situation, that you are in your gynaecology theatre and preparing to perform the procedure. Describe each step of the procedure. This shows the examiner that you are competent, safe and confident. Practice describing each procedure to your revision buddy.

Take the opportunity to go to a urogynaecology list before the MRCOG Part 3 exam so that you can familiarise yourself with common urogynaecological procedures if it has been a while since operating on one of these lists. Ask the scrub nurse to talk you through assembling the endoscopes.

MODULE 3: POST-OPERATIVE CARE

Candidate instructions

This task is a structured viva:

- Information gathering
- Applied clinical knowledge
- Patient safety
- Communication with patients

A 43-year-old woman underwent a total laparoscopic hysterectomy for symptomatic endometriosis 7 days previously. She is admitted with right-sided abdominal pain. On examination, her temperature is 38.5°C, her heart rate 105 beats per minute, respiratory rate is 18 and her blood pressure is 135/80 mmHg. The surgical sites are beginning to heal. She has normal heart and chest sounds, but there is diffuse mild tenderness in the abdomen with normal bowel sounds. There is severe right renal angle tenderness.

You have 10 minutes to answer a series of questions from the examiner regarding the management of this woman.

Examiner instructions

This is a structured VIVA. You should ask the candidate the questions on your mark sheet. You can prompt the candidate if necessary, but this requirement should be reflected in the global marks awarded.

Questions to be asked:

1. What diagnosis are you considering and why?
2. How would initially manage and investigate this patient?
3. What is your management strategy now?
4. Describe the course of the ureter and explain where the likely injury points could be?
5. What would you do after care has been taken over the urologists?

Marking

Communication with colleagues
- Consultants/senior gynaecologists should be called appropriately.
- The management plan should involve colleagues from other specialities as appropriate.

Information gathering

- Arranges appropriate investigations for a sepsis and possible ureteric obstruction or injury.
- The intravenous pyelogram should be interpreted correctly.

Patient safety

- The candidate should recognise the limitations of the clinical abilities and call senior colleagues appropriately.
- The sepsis pathway should be followed.
- The candidate should demonstrate an understanding of the role of clinical governance in relation to post-operative complications.

Applied clinical knowledge

- The candidate considers pyelonephritis, right ureteric injury and obstruction as part of the differential diagnosis.
- The candidate should have knowledge of the route of the ureter and the areas in which it is most likely to be damaged during hysterectomy.
- An appropriate and well-thought-out management plan should be given at each stage.

What diagnosis are you considering and why?

Pyelonephritis or right ureteral obstruction/injury.

The presentation is what you would expect for pyelonephritis but given the history of a recent hysterectomy, the candidate should appreciate that there is a risk of obstruction or injury to the ureter. The history of endometriosis is a risk factor for ureteric injury.

How would you initially investigate this patient?

Initial management should consist of beginning the sepsis pathway (catheter, blood cultures, IV fluids, IV antibiotics, lactate, FBC, CRP, U&Es, lactate and oxygen). Given the suspected diagnosis, the on-call consultant and/or consultant who performed the case should be informed. There should be an appropriate investigation for an obstructed or damaged ureter such as an intravenous pyelogram, but a CT scan with intravenous contrast could also be diagnostic. If you are uncertain, a consultant radiologist can give the best modality for imaging.

What is your management strategy now?

If not already done, the on-call consultant and/or consultant who performed the case should be informed. The on-call urologist will need to be called unless the gynaecology consultant is qualified to perform repairs independently. In the event of unexpected complications, it is better to seek expert help even if the gynaecology consultant is qualified. They will look to stent the lumen or, if transected, end-to-end anastomosis at the pelvic brim while damage near the bladder edge is better repaired using ureteric reimplantation into the bladder using a psoas hitch or bladder flap to relieve tension on the repair. There is a duty of candour, and an apology should be given to the patient – usually by the consultant responsible for the case.

Describe the course of the ureter and explain where the likely injury points could be

The ureters arise from the pelvis of the kidney and descend into the pelvis over the psoas muscle to reach the brim of the pelvis. At this point, they go anterior to the common iliac vessels. At the level of the pelvic brim, the ureter can be damaged during ligation of the ovarian vessels .Beyond the pelvic brim, the ureters pass down the side of the pelvis until and run under the uterine arteries ('water under the bridge'). At this point, the ureter is between 1 and 3 cm lateral to the cervix and is the most common site of injury during hysterectomy. This can happen when the cardinal ligaments and uterine arteries are clamped, cut and ligated. The ureters then run into the back on the bladder and anterior to the vagina and inserted into the bladder trigone. The ureters can be damaged when running anterior to the vagina when the vaginal cuff is ligated.

What would you do after care has been taken over by the urologist?

An incident form needs to be submitted and serious case review held to see if any lessons can be learnt to prevent this happening in the future. The patient should be followed up regularly, not only while she is an inpatient but also in gynaecology outpatients.

MODULE 4: ANTENATAL CARE

Candidate instructions

This station is a role-play station and will assess your abilities to take a booking history for a woman who has a twin gestation and to provide a plan of care for on-going pregnancy. You will be assessed using the following domains:

- Patient safety
- Communication with patients and their relatives
- Information gathering
- Applied clinical knowledge

You will see Nasreen Akhtar, a 26-year-old woman who has just found out that she is pregnant for the first time. She has just attended for her dating scan, which shows that she is pregnant with twins. Her dating scan report is as follows:

Nasreen Akhtar
DOB 23/07/1991
Daye of ultrasound examination: 23/10/2017
T/A ultrasound findings:
There are two viable intrauterine pregnancies seen.

Lambda sign is seen at the membrane placental interface suggestive of a DCDA pregnancy.

Foetal heart activity is seen in both foetuses.

The gestation age has been determined by measurement of the CRL 51 mm – 11 + 3/40 gestation.

The NT has not been measured today.

You will have 10 minutes to take an obstetric history, discuss twin pregnancy and organise a plan for the on-going pregnancy.

Simulated patient instructions

You are Nasreen Akhtar, a 26-year-old office administrator who is 11 weeks into your first pregnancy. You and your partner had been trying to conceive for the past 12 months and you are delighted to have found out that you will be having twins. You are unaware of any of the risks that are associated with twin pregnancy and become very concerned when these are communicated to you.

You have mild asthma and eczema. You have never required hospital treatment for these conditions. You take salbutamol inhalers when required and use emollients for your eczema. You previously had a diagnostic laparoscopy for pelvic pain, which you were told was normal. You are not allergic to anything and do not smoke or drink alcohol.

You would like to have Down's syndrome screening.

If not covered by the candidate, questions that you could ask include the following:

- What kind of twins am I having?
- Will it be two girls or two boys or a mixture?
- Will I be able to have Down's syndrome screening?
- Will I require further ultrasound scans during this pregnancy?
- When will I be delivered?
- How will I be delivered?

Marking

Patient safety

- Knowledgeable regarding twin gestations and provides accurate information regarding chorionicity.
- Provides a suitable plan of management for the rest of the DCDA pregnancy.
- Arranges Down's syndrome screening on request of the patient by referral to the foetal medicine specialist.

Communication with patients and their relatives

- Demonstrates good communication skills during history taking.
- Acknowledges the patient's concerns and anxieties.
- Explains the risks of twin pregnancy at a pace at which the patient can understand and encourages patient to ask questions if they have any queries.
- Ensures the patient understands and is content with the plan for the rest of the pregnancy.

- Avoidance of medical jargon throughout.
- Answers questions posed by the patient in a clear manner.

Information gathering

- Demonstrates a clear structure when taking an obstetric history.
- Listens to the patient attentively and allows good flow of information.
- Interprets the scan findings correctly.
- Assesses the wish of the patient regarding mode of delivery.
- Attempts to find out further information regarding the previous C/S at the neighbouring hospital.

Applied clinical knowledge

- Demonstrates the knowledge of twin pregnancy.
- Understands the risks of twin pregnancy and how to monitor for these risks.
- Demonstrates the knowledge of management of twin pregnancy.

Examiner notes

- In this clinical scenario, the candidate should take a concise obstetric history. This should include POH, PMH, PSH, DH, allergy history, social history.
- The candidate should be able to explain the meaning of DCDA twins without the use of jargon – two placentas and two sacs, one for each baby
- The candidate will describe the risks of twin pregnancy to the patient. These include the following:
  - Anaemia
  - Pregnancy-induced hypertension and pre-eclampsia
  - Gestational diabetes
  - Haemorrhage – abruption, praevia, PPH
  - Preterm delivery (<32/40) 10% prevalence
  - Selective IUGR (>20% discordance) 11%–20% prevalence
  - Screening for trisomy 21 and 80%–90% accurate only with NT screen
- The concerns and anxieties of the patient should be acknowledged and appropriate reassurance should be provided such that the patient is made aware that the risks are present but the majority of twin pregnancies are uncomplicated.
- The candidate will provide a plan for the rest of the pregnancy in a manner such that the patient understands what will happen next. The plan should include the following:
  - Offer Down's syndrome screening by referral to local foetal medicine specialist for measurement of NT
  - Booking bloods
  - An extra Hb at 20 weeks gestation to monitor for anaemia
  - 28/40 bloods
  - Glucose tolerance testing at 26–28/40
  - Growth scans every 4 weeks from 20 weeks gestation to monitor for selective IUGR

- Start low dose aspirin as nulliparous and multiple pregnancy
- Aim delivery at 37 weeks
- The candidate should provide information regarding mode of delivery. Explaining that this will be determined by the presentation of the first twin and that the delivery will be at around 37 weeks gestation.
- Once the plan has been finalised, the candidate should check understanding with the patient and ensure that the patient is satisfied with the plan for her on-going pregnancy.

Revision notes

A quick obstetric history should be taken from the patient. It is important to check the patient's knowledge of twins and then provide an explanation of chorionicity with an avoidance of jargon. Simply, a DCDA twin pregnancy is just as if the patient has two singletons. Remember that Down's syndrome screening is possible by assessing NT but is not as accurate when compared with combined screening in singleton pregnancies.

Your knowledge of twin gestation risks and management is being examined but as this is the Part 3 MRCOG, the manner in which you explain these risks and the steps that will be taken in the management to identify any abnormalities with the pregnancy is just as important as your knowledge.

Lastly, this station is an ideal example in which your knowledge must still be sharp when you prepare for the Part 3 MRCOG. Although this is a professional examination, your ability to explain difficult concepts will be enhanced by a solid foundation of clinical knowledge.

Further reading: NICE multiple pregnancy guideline.

MODULE 5: MATERNAL MEDICINE

Candidate instructions

This is a simulated patient assessing the following:

- Communication with patients
- Information gathering
- Patient safety
- Applied clinical knowledge

Emma Hardy, a 28-year-old woman has come for an early booking appointment. She is 8/40 by dates with a BMI of 24. The midwife says she is a known epileptic and reports feeling nauseous.

You have 10 minutes to

1. Take a short history.
2. Give a specific management plan during pregnancy.
3. Answer any patient questions.

Simulated patient instructions

You are Emma Hardy, a 28-year-old police officer in her first pregnancy. You were diagnosed with epilepsy when you were 8 years old. The condition has been stable and your last fit was 6 months ago. People that have seen your fit describe you falling to the floor with jerking of your arms and legs for around 1–3 minutes. Often you bite the inside of your mouth or tongue. Afterwards you feel tired and confused.

Your last menstrual period was 8 weeks ago. You have a dating scan arranged in 4 weeks time. You having been feeling increasingly nauseous and have vomited twice. You have not taken anything for nausea and vomiting.

You are currently taking lamotrigine 100 mg once a day and are under the care of the neurologist. You have no other medical problems and have never had any surgery. You do not smoke, drink or take recreational drugs.

If not covered by the candidate, the following questions may be useful:

- How will epilepsy affect my pregnancy?
- What care will I get during pregnancy?
- What should I do if vomit after taking my medication?
- Will I be able to have the usual pain relief during labour?
- Will I be able to breast-feed my baby while taking my epilepsy medication?

Marking

Communication with patient

- Adequate introduction, good body language and eye contact.
- Able to describe the impact of epilepsy on pregnancy while avoiding medical jargon.
- Give the patient information in manageable amounts.
- Addresses concerns of patient in an empathetic manner.

Information gathering

- The candidate should take a relevant antenatal history (see "Examiner notes").
- Uses open questions and signposting to direct the consultation.

Applied clinical knowledge

- The candidate should demonstrate knowledge of the impact of epilepsy on pregnancy and the foetus.
- The candidate should formulate an appropriate antenatal management for a woman with epilepsy, which should involve antenatal care with specialist epilepsy team.

Safety

- The candidate should emphasise the importance of taking their epilepsy medication and not adjust the dose unless they have consulted with their health professional.

- The candidate should check that the woman is taking high dose folic acid.
- The candidate should know that pethidine is not recommended in women with epilepsy.

Examiner notes

History

A competent candidate will gather information quickly by guiding the patient with open questions. Below is an example framework that can be used to take an antenatal history:

- Presenting complaint
  - What seems to be the problem? How can I help you?
  - Systematic enquiry (in this case, it is important to establish how, what type and how often the seizures are)
- Antenatal care to date
  - How has your pregnancy been so far?
  - Have your scans been normal?
- Past obstetrics history
  - Have you had any previous pregnancies?
  - Were there any problems?
  - Were they normal deliveries?
- Past medical/surgical history
  - Do you have any medical problems?
  - Have you had any operations in the past?
- Drug history
  - Are you taking any medications at the moment? (folic acid dose, epileptic medication and compliance should be elicited)
  - Do you have any drug allergies?
- Family history
  - Do any illnesses run in the family?
- Social history
  - Do you drink or smoke?
  - Do you take any recreational drugs?
  - Screening for domestic abuse
    - Have you felt threatened by anyone?
    - Do you feel scared by anyone?

Management

Ideally, advice about epilepsy and pregnancy should be given preconception, but half of pregnancies in women with epilepsy are unplanned. Once pregnant, it is important to manage the complications of early pregnancy, such as vomiting, which may reduce the levels of anti-epileptic drugs leading to exacerbation.

How will epilepsy affect my pregnancy?

When counselling women with medical conditions in pregnancy it is often useful to break down into effects on the baby and effects on the woman:

For the baby

There is an increased risk of abnormalities in babies born to women taking certain types of epilepsy medication. Sodium valproate is the drug that is most associated with these abnormalities and consideration should be given to changing it before or during pregnancy. The most common abnormalities associated with epilepsy medication include spina bifida, facial cleft or heart abnormalities. Taking folic acid reduces this risk and should be given at high dose (5 mg). Ideally, this should be given 3 months preconception.

For the woman

Around a third of women will have seizure deterioration in pregnancy. There is also an increased risk of sudden death particularly for those that suffer grand mal seizures. It is important to reduce the risk of seizures and this can be done by ensuring the patients are well rested and take their medications. Given the risks associated with epilepsy medication, it is not surprising that many women stop their medication once they have found out they are pregnant. It is important to emphasise that the risk of the medication is small, but the risk of stopping the medication poses a serious risk to both the woman and the baby.

What should I do if vomit after taking my medication?

If within 40 minutes, or they can see the tablet within the vomit, then they should retake their medication. If they are having trouble with nausea and vomiting, they should contact their GP, midwife or epilepsy specialist.

What care will I get during pregnancy?

The patient can be told to expect to have more frequent antenatal visits with a designated epilepsy care team with both obstetric and epilepsy/neurology specialists. In addition to the anomaly scan, growth scans from 26 to 28/40 can be arranged if taking antiepileptic's or having seizures. High dose folic acid 5 mg/day should be prescribed until at least the end of the first trimester. Routine monitoring of antiepileptic drug levels is not recommended. Women should be provided with information about the UK Epilepsy and Pregnancy register.

What pain relief can I take during labour?

The usual range of pain relief in labour is available for women with epilepsy except for Pethidine. Pethidine is not recommended, because in high doses, it is associated with seizures.

Will I be able to breast feed my baby while taking my epilepsy medication?

Small amounts will pass through the breast milk, but this is not considered harmful. In fact the baby will be used to having the medication and maybe a little jittery if they are formula fed.

MODULE 6: MANAGEMENT OF LABOUR

Candidate instructions

This station is a role-play station and will assess your abilities to counsel a woman who has been found to be breech presentation in the first stage of labour. You will be assessed using the following domains:

- Patient safety
- Communication with patients and their relatives
- Information gathering
- Applied clinical knowledge

You are the labour ward registrar and have been asked by your consultant to counsel a patient, Ellen Smith, regarding her delivery. Mrs Smith attended the hospital as she had started having contractions 4 hours ago and the pain was getting to be too much to manage at home. Your consultant has performed a transabdominal ultrasound scan, which has shown that the foetus has an extended breech presentation. Your consultant has been called away to manage a gynaecology emergency. The patient has been found to be 3cm dilated and was otherwise low risk during her pregnancy. The only ultrasound scans that she had undergone were her dating scan and her 20-week anomaly scan. She was hoping to have a normal vaginal delivery. She is currently 39+2 weeks pregnant. The CTG is normal.

You will have 10 minutes to take an obstetric history and discuss the mode of delivery.

Simulated patient instructions

You are Ellen Smith, a 26-year-old primary school teacher who is 39 weeks into your first pregnancy. You have been hoping for a normal vaginal delivery throughout your pregnancy and have been reading books to help to manage your contractions and labour. You have had no issues during your pregnancy and are very annoyed when you are told that your baby is breech. You want to know why the breech presentation was not identified prior to you attending in labour and why you are being counselled about having a C/S.

With effective counselling, you agree to have a C/S but you want to know what will happen next and who will be in the operating theatre. You also wish to know how long you will be in hospital and how you will feel after the operation is completed.

If not covered by the candidate, questions that you could ask include the following:

- Why was the breech presentation not picked up before?
- Why do I need to have a C/S?
- Why has the consultant not bothered to tell me this himself?
- What will happen next if I am to have a C/S?
- Is my partner allowed with me in theatre?
- Who else will be with me in theatre?
- How long will the operation take?

- How will I feel after the C/S is finished?
- How long will I be in hospital?

Marking

Patient safety
- Knowledgeable regarding breech presentation and the risks and benefits for C/S and breech vaginal delivery.
- Demonstrates that the breech C/S should be performed without delay.

Communication with patients and their relatives
- Demonstrates good communication skills during history taking.
- Acknowledges the patient's anger and frustration.
- Apologises for the clinical situation and that the consultant had to leave.
- Addresses the emotions of the patient rather than taking a pragmatic approach.
- Offers the option of breech vaginal delivery and emergency C/S but recommends C/S as the safest mode of delivery.
- Explains the need for C/S in a clear manner.
- Explains ongoing management so that the patient is aware of what will happen next.

Information gathering
- Demonstrates a clear structure when taking an obstetric history.
- Gathers the patient's views and opinions.

Applied clinical knowledge
- Demonstrates knowledge of breech presentation in labour.
- Understands the mode of delivery options available.
- Demonstrates understanding of what will happen in the operating theatre and what will happen to the patient postnatally.

Examiner notes

- In this clinical scenario, the candidate should take a concise obstetric history. This should include POH, PMH, PSH, DH, allergy history, social history and when they last ate or drank.
- The candidate should listen to the patients concerns that the breech presentation was not identified without incriminating the community midwife. They should explain that breech presentation can be difficult to determine on abdominal examination alone, and this clinical situation does occur from time to time.
- The frustrations of the patient that the consultant has had to attend to another patient should be listened to attentively and acknowledged.
- The candidate should demonstrate empathy and apologise that the circumstances are as they are.
- The candidate does not interrupt the patient and demonstrates evidence of active listening.

- The options for delivery should be provided with an adequate explanation of the risks with breech vaginal delivery, which include the following:
  - An increase in the short-term morbidity of the baby
  - Risks of entrapment of the after-coming head
- The risks of emergency C/S should also be discussed.
  - Bleeding
  - Infection
  - Thromboembolism
  - Pain
  - Damage to other intra-abdominal structures
  - Cut or marks to the baby
  - Need for blood transfusion or repair to any damaged structures
- Overall, the recommendation here would to have an emergency C/S.
- The candidates should be able to answer the patient's queries in a confident manner.
  - Completion of consent form.
  - Anaesthetic review.
  - Blood tests for Group and Save and FBC.
  - Transfer to the theatre for a category II C/S.
  - The partner will be allowed in theatre.
  - There will be two surgeons, three theatre team members, the midwife, the anaesthetist and the neonatal doctor.
  - The patient will be in hospital for 2–3 days and will make a full recovery in 6 weeks time.

Revision notes

In this scenario, your ability to manage an angry patient is being assessed. Try not to interrupt the patient as they are making their thoughts known to you. Calmly apologise about what has happened. This does not admit fault on behalf of the community midwife or consultant but does acknowledge that you are sorry for the situation that the patient finds herself in. Good candidates will be able to appease the patient quite quickly by using effective communication skills to ensure that the patient feels that they are being listened to. Adopting a solution-based approach with an angry patient is unlikely to be successful. Instead try to acknowledge emotions and empathise.

MODULE 7: MANAGEMENT OF DELIVERY

Candidate instructions

This station is with a simulated patient and will assess the following domains:

- Communication with colleagues
- Information gathering
- Applied clinical knowledge
- Patient safety

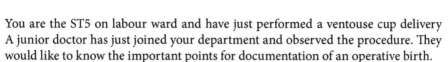

You are the ST5 on labour ward and have just performed a ventouse cup delivery A junior doctor has just joined your department and observed the procedure. They would like to know the important points for documentation of an operative birth.

You have 10 minutes in which to describe the following:

1. Why is good documentation important for operative delivery
2. The principles of good documentation for operative birth
3. Support of the trainees' further learning

Simulated trainee instructions

You are a foundation year 2 doctor starting your first placement in obstetrics and gynaecology. It is a career that interests you and you have attended an introductory course and know the principles of a forceps and ventouse delivery. Although the course went into the technical details of operative vaginal delivery, it did not cover the documentation. You are aware that delivery of babies is an area of high litigation and have been told that meticulous documentation is important to convey a high standard of care. You cannot think of any other reasons why good documentation is important.

If not covered by the candidate, questions that you could ask include the following:

- Why is good documentation important?
- Which parts of the management before the procedure need to be documented?
- What else should you document about the procedure?

Marking

Communication with colleagues
- Appropriate introduction.
- There should be a clear structure to the delivery of teaching.
- Encourages learning, discussion and questions with appropriate verbal and non-verbal communication.

Information gathering
- Checks the existing knowledge of the candidate.
- Confirms understanding at appropriate intervals during teaching.

Applied clinical knowledge
- The competent candidate will know why meticulous documentation is important.
- The candidate should demonstrate a clear understanding of the important points to document as suggested in the examiner's notes section.

Safety
- The candidate should demonstrate knowledge of the prerequisites of operative vaginal delivery through teaching of correct documentation.

• The trainee should have a clear idea of what points should be documented. They should be given a safe learning plan. For example, the trainee could be directed to the proforma within the greentop guideline and should be advised to have a senior colleague check their documentation after their next procedure.

Examiner notes

Good documentation is important for clear communication to colleagues, education, audit and clinical governance. Proformas can be a useful way of ensuring thorough documentation. An example proforma for operative vaginal birth can be found within the RCOG green-top guideline for operative birth.

Areas that should be included for documentation about operative birth are as follows:

1. Date, time, name and position
2. Management prior to delivery
   a. Indication for delivery
   b. Foetal condition
      i. CTG
      ii. Liquor
   c. Analgesia
   d. Abdominal and vaginal examination findings including the following:
      i. Station
      ii. Engagement
      iii. Position
      iv. Caput
      v. Moulding
   e. Consent
3. Procedure details
   a. Person performing procedure (± supervision) with experience level
   b. Bladder care
   c. Rotation of head
   d. Instrument(s) used and order if sequential instruments used
   e. Ease of application
   f. Descent
   g. Number of pulls
   h. Foetal heart rate
   i. Episiotomy performed
4. Post-procedure details
   a. Condition of the baby
      i. Cord pH
      ii. APGAR
   b. Estimated blood loss
   c. Perineal assessment
   d. Thromboembolic risk
   e. Swab and instrument count

MODULE 8: POSTPARTUM MANAGEMENT

Candidate instructions

This station is a structured VIVA and will assess your abilities to answer questions surrounding the perinatal mental health. You will be assessed using the following domains:

- Patient safety
- Communication with colleagues
- Information gathering
- Applied clinical knowledge

You are the registrar on-call on labour ward, it is the weekend. A midwife on the postnatal floor has asked whether you can attend to review a patient that she is very concerned about. The patient had an emergency C/S 3 days ago. She is still an in-patient because the baby is receiving antibiotic therapy for neonatal sepsis. This is the patient's first delivery. The midwife is concerned that the patient is acting withdrawn and not paying a lot of attention to the baby.

You will have 10 minutes to answer questions regarding your assessment and management of this patient. You will be assessed according to your ability in answering the questions and the amount of prompting that you require.

Marking

Patient safety

- Understands the risks that are posed in perinatal mental health conditions and that maternal and neonatal safety are paramount.
- Escalates to seniors appropriately.
- Arranges onward referral to other medical specialities (psychiatry) appropriately.

Communication with colleagues

- Provides clear and structured answers.
- Evidence of methodical approaches to tackling problems and is able to communicate management plans.

Information gathering

- Understands important factors within the history to gather to aid in the diagnosis and management of perinatal mental health disorders.
- Able to compile a panel of investigations to ensure that there is no organic cause of acute confusional state.

Applied clinical knowledge

- Demonstrates knowledge of perinatal mental health disorders.
- Able to apply knowledge such that an effective management plan can be implemented.

Examiner notes

Ask the questions below to the candidate in the sequence provided.

1. When you see the patient you believe that she is suffering with baby blues. The midwife believes the woman has postnatal depression. What are the differences between baby blues and postnatal depression?
   * Characteristics of baby blues
     – Affects up to 50% of mothers.
     – Due to hormonal changes shortly after delivery.
     – Characteristically, symptoms are experienced 3–5 days after delivery.
     – Symptoms include feelings of irritability, tearfulness, anxiety.
     – Short lived.
     – Requires supportive therapy only.
   * Characteristics of postnatal depression
     – Affects 10% of women.
     – Usually, the onset of symptoms is 2–8 weeks after delivery.
     – Symptoms include anhedonia, lack of energy, insomnia, lack of appetite, early morning wakening, feelings of hopelessness.
     – May need formal cognitive behavioural therapy or antidepressants for treatment.

2. The next day, events have turned for the worse; the midwife tells you that the woman is now behaving more strangely. She appears to be hallucinating and is accusing the midwives of trying to harm her and her baby. You now think she may have developed puerperal psychosis. What are the features of puerperal psychosis?
   * Affects 1 in 1000 women after delivery and is a medical emergency
   * Symptoms
     – Hallucinations –usually auditory
     – Delusions – fixed held false beliefs
     – Feelings of elation
     – Flight of ideas
     – Low mood
     – Loss of inhibitions
     – Feelings of fear

3. What are the risk factors for the development of puerperal psychosis?
   * Personal history of puerperal psychosis after a previous pregnancy
   * Family history of mental health illnesses (especially puerperal psychosis)
   * Traumatic birth
   * Personal history of bipolar affective disorder or schizophrenia

4. How will you assess this patient now?
   * Perform a metal health assessment. In particular, look for the following:
     – Engagement
     – Eye contact
     – Any suggestion of reaction to external stimuli that are not present

- Perform a risk assessment for continuing maternal and neonatal safety. In particular, enquire about thoughts of deliberate self harm, suicide and infanticide.
- Find out about any delusional beliefs.
- Assess maternal observations.
- If possible carry out a full examination including a neurological examination.
- Try to rule out any organic causes of acute confusional state given that she is now 4 days post C/S such as the following:
  - Infection
  - Anaemia
  - Electrolyte disturbances
  - Stroke
- The candidate may remark that ruling these causes of acute confusional state may not possible if the patient is acutely psychotic.

5. How will you manage her now?
  - Simple practical steps
    - Nurse in a single room if possible.
    - Nurse close to the midwifery station.
    - Do not remove baby away from mother unless clear risks identified to the baby as doing so would likely cause deterioration in the patient's mental state.
    - Offer support to the midwifery team.
  - The candidate should comment that this is an emergency situation, and there are genuine risks for the patient, her baby and the staff.
  - Inform the consultant of the events.
  - If causes of acute confusional state can be ruled out, refer to on-call psychiatric services.
  - Ideal referral location would be a specialised mother and baby unit.

Revision notes

Perinatal mental health is rightly a hot topic for RCOG. It is often neglected by MRCOG Part 3 candidates. Ensure that you are well versed in perinatal mental health conditions as it could potentially crop up in a variety of different guises in the OSCE circuit.

This type of station assesses your clinical knowledge and how you can apply it to a particularly challenging scenario whilst keeping patient safety in the forefront of your mind. Additionally, the examiner will be assessing how you can provide a clear structure to your answers as the clinical situation evolves. Many knowledgeable candidates struggle with constructing structured answers and often list answers off in a scattergun manner. What is required is a moment's thought after each question, to gain composure and a few seconds to think before delivering the answer. This ability to take your time is difficult to display in the OSCE circuit, but if achieved can lead to the delivery of a mature and methodical answer.

MODULE 9: GENERAL GYNAECOLOGY

Candidate instructions

This station is with a simulated patient and will assess the following domains:

- Information gathering
- Communication with patients
- Applied clinical knowledge
- Patient safety

You have been asked to see a 35-year-old, social worker, Ms Tracey Hardy, who presented with irregular and heavy menstrual bleeding with a BMI of 36. When she was seen previously an endometrial biopsy was taken and a pelvic ultrasound was organised. The results are shown as follows:

Pathology report

Patient name: Tracey Hardy
   DOB: 01/03/1983 (Age: 35)
   Clinical details: heavy menstrual bleeding
   Specimen: pipelle biopsy
   Gross description: Multiple pieces of tan-red tissue mixed with haemorrhagic material
   Microscopic diagnosis: Endometrial hyperplasia without atypia

Radiology report

Patient name: Tracey Hardy
   DOB: 01/03/1983 (Age: 35)
   Clinical details: heavy menstrual bleeding
   Scan performed: transabdominal and transvaginal
   Impression: 9 cm anteverted uterus, 10mm endometrial thickness, normal ovaries, no fluid in the pouch of Douglas.

You have 10 minutes to do the following:

1. Take a relevant history.
2. Explain the findings of the two investigations.
3. Formulate and explain a management plan to the patient.
4. Answer any questions the patient has.

Simulated patient instructions

You are Tracey Hardy, a 35-year-old social worker. For the past 5 years, you have had increasingly heavy menstrual bleeding, which can last up to 9 days. You need to change your pad 10 times a day when the bleeding is at its worst and have taken time off work because of the period pain and bleeding. Over the past 12 months, you have also developed intermenstrual spotting. Your periods are regular.

You have had partners in the past but are currently not seeing anyone. You have never tried to get pregnant but would like to start a family when you meet the right person. You are concerned about what hyperplasia means to your fertility.

Your GP gave you Tranexamic acid to help with the bleeding, but there was no improvement. You did not take the offer of hormonal treatment by the GP, because you heard that you would put on weight. However, you will consider oral hormonal treatment if your concerns are discussed and the risks of the hyperplasia are given. You will not consider an intrauterine device under any circumstances, as you do not like the idea of something 'being inside you'.

Your general health is good and you had your appendix out when you were 10 years old. Your smear tests have been normal. You drink on special occasions and smoke 10 cigarettes a day because you have a stressful job. There is no family history of note.

If not covered by the candidate, the following questions may be helpful:

- Do I have cancer/what is my risk of cancer?
- How does this affect my fertility?
- How long will I have to take the medication?
- How will I be followed up?

Marking

Information gathering
- The candidate should take a relevant gynaecological history (see "Examiner notes").
- They should show the ability to interpret the histology and ultrasound report.

Communication with patients
- Uses appropriate warning shot(s) before telling the woman there is hyperplasia.
- Gives the patient information in manageable amounts avoiding jargon.
- Responds appropriately to patient concerns.

Applied clinical knowledge
- The risk of progression should be conveyed with accurate numbers.
- The candidate should be able to use the history and investigations to formulate a management plan in line with RCOG guidelines. This should include lifestyle modifications.

Patient safety
- The candidate should explain that the best chance of regression is with the LNG-IUS, but a negotiated treatment with oral medication or weight loss and observation of 6 months is acceptable.
- There should be an understanding of the RCOG treatment pathway with appropriate short-term and long-term follow-ups.

Examiner notes

History taking

The key things to find out in this history should include that she is nulliparous and desires a family in the future; other treatments that have been given/not given and why; medical history that affects her risk and lifestyle factors such as smoking. An example history may look like as follows:

- Presenting complaint (How can I help you? If it were the first meeting):
  - Systematic enquiry
    - Menstrual – do you have heavy bleeding or tell me about you bleeding?
      - Regular– anovulatory cycles are risk for hyperplasia
      - IMB, PCB
  - Any previous treatments?
  - Have your smear tests been normal?
  - Any previous pregnancies?
  - Any plans to get pregnant in the future?
  - Any previous infections/PID?
- Past medical/surgical history
  - Do you have any medical problems?
  - Have you had any operations in the past?
- Drug history
  - Are you taking any medications at the moment including contraceptives?
  - Do you have any drug allergies?
- Family history
  - Do any illnesses run in the family?
- Social history
  - Do you drink or smoke?
  - Do you take any recreational drugs?

Management

Endometrial hyperplasia occurs due to oestrogenic stimulation of the endometrium without appropriate regulation from progesterone. The known risk factors reflect this and include raised BMI, oestrogen secreting tumours (e.g. granulosa cell tumours), drug-induced endometrial stimulation (e.g. tamoxifen) and anovulatory cycles caused by polycystic ovarian syndrome and perimenopause.

Endometrial hyperplasia can be classified into hyperplasia without atypia and atypical hyperplasia. For hyperplasia without atypia, the risk of progression to endometrial cancer is <5% over 20 years. Most cases of hyperplasia without atypia will regress spontaneously, but women need to be informed that treatment with progestogens give a much higher rate of regression.

Management of hyperplasia without atypia is as follows:

- Address reversible risk factors – In this case, it is advice about obesity but in other patients this could be modification of HRT regimens, tamoxifen and treating anovulation.

- First line medical treatment would be the LNG-IUS, but as this is not acceptable to the patient, she should have second line treatment, which would be oral progestogens or observation with weight loss. Given her symptoms of heavy menstrual bleeding, progestogens are the obvious choice. Third line treatment would be total hysterectomy±BSO, but this is not suitable due to her wish to retain fertility in the future.
- A repeat endometrial biopsy should be performed in 6 months.
- Further management will depend on whether the repeat endometrial biopsy shows regression, persistence or progression.
    - Progression should have total hysterectomy + BSO.
    - Persistence with progestogen treatment should consider total hysterectomy + BSO those observed should start progestogen treatment.
    - If there is regression, then a repeat biopsy should be done in another 6 months. If the subsequent biopsy is normal, the patient should have annual screening as this patient has a BMI ≥35 and will not accept the LNG-IUS as treatment.

Further reading: RCOG greentop guideline on management of hyperplasia.

MODULE 10: SUBFERTILITY

Candidate instructions

This station is a role-play station and will assess your abilities to explain the diagnosis and treatment of Kayleigh Madden who is a 28-year-old nurse. She has never been pregnant before and her partner has never fathered any children. You are seeing her in the infertility clinic for follow-up after she had baseline fertility investigations. She had been trying to conceive for the past 3 years. The investigations are as follows:

Female hormone profile
- FSH 4.3
- LH 5.1
- Estradiol 234
- Rubella IgG positive
- Mid luteal progesterone 32

Ultrasound pelvis
Normal uterus, endometrium and adnexae

Hysterosalpingogram
- Normal filling of endometrial cavity
- Fill and spill of bilateral fallopian tubes

Seminal fluid analysis
- Count 6 million/mL
- Volume 3.1 mL

- Motility 23%
- Progressive motility 12%
- Normal morphology 2%

You will be assessed using the following domains:

- Patient safety
- Communication with patients and their relatives
- Information gathering
- Applied clinical knowledge

You will have 10 minutes to explain to Kayleigh the results of the tests and to inform her of the best course of management.

Simulated patient instructions

You are Kayleigh Madden, a 28-year-old nurse who has been trying for a baby for the past 3 years. You are married to Rob, who is unable to attend the clinic appointment with you today as he is at work as a chef. You were initially referred by your GP 3 months ago to the fertility clinic.

When you are told that Rob has had an abnormal semen analysis, you are shocked. You become upset and tearful that you may not be able to have children. You need to be reassured that there are treatments available that will allow you to become pregnant before you stop being upset. After this, you would like to know more about the ICSI treatment that has been suggested.

If not covered by the candidate, questions that you could ask include the following:

- What is the possible cause for why Rob has low sperm concentration?
- Is there anything that Rob can do to improve his sperm count?
- Would it have made any difference if we were referred earlier by the GP?
- Can you tell me what happens in ICSI treatment?
- Roughly, how successful is ICSI treatment?
- How much will the ICSI treatment cost?
- What will happen now?

Marking

Patient safety
- Conveys accurate information regarding the diagnosis and treatment.
- Admits that they are not sure rather than trying to appear knowledgeable.

Communication with patients and their relatives
- Acknowledges the patient's disappointment regarding the diagnosis of male infertility.
- Shows empathy towards the patient's situation.
- Demonstrates effective communication skills to manage the patient's emotions.
- Explains the diagnosis clearly.

- Explains the concept of ICSI treatment whilst avoiding jargons.
- Conveys management plan in a manner which is easy to digest.

Information gathering
- Interprets investigation results correctly.
- Gathers information regarding Rob and how he may improve his semen analysis (e.g. quitting smoking, limit alcohol and caffeine intake).
- Gathers information regarding patients baseline understanding of ICSI treatment and male infertility.

Applied clinical knowledge
- Makes the correct diagnosis of male infertility.
- Answers the patient's questions correctly.
- Demonstrates a clear understanding of NICE fertility guidelines.
- Demonstrates a clear understanding of ICSI treatment.

Examiner notes

- The candidate should find out what the patient knows of the clinical situation.
- An appropriate warning shot should be given with the diagnosis of male factor infertility delivered soon after.
- Time should be given to the patient to digest the bad news.
- An explanation of how male factor infertility causes infertility should be given.
- The candidate should answer the questions asked by the patient accurately.
- A repeat SFA should be organised.
- The candidate could enquire about the male partner's social history – smoking status, alcohol and caffeine intake.
- There would likely to have been no difference in the semen analysis result, if the GP referral had been made earlier. Also the ovarian reserve is normal.
- ICSI treatment should be described with the avoidance of jargon, and a diagram could be drawn to illustrate the treatment concept.
- It is likely the candidate may not know the success rate of ICSI or where the patient would be referred to. If this is the case, then the candidate should admit that they are unsure and that they would seek appropriate advice from the infertility team.
- The success rate of a 28-year-old undergoing ICSI treatment is roughly 35%. The candidate may mention that they would refer to the local infertility unit or team for funding application and assessment.
- Written information could be provided.

Revision notes

Although subfertility is a subspeciality of gynaecology, you will be expected to know basic concepts of treatment if asked by patients. So a sound basic knowledge is required. The aim of this station is to assess your ability to break the news of male factor infertility and display your effective communications skills to move the consultation on to discuss the management.

Remember to not pretend to know about aspects of O&G that you are not familiar with. You may not be familiar with success rates of ICSI treatment, where the patient will need to be referred or the funding rules and this is within reason for the MRCOG. What is not reasonable is to provide false information as this is unsafe practice and will be easily detected by the examiners. Instead just admit that you are unsure but can find out more information from your seniors.

MODULE 11: SEXUAL AND REPRODUCTIVE HEALTH

Candidate instructions

This station is with a simulated patient and will assess the following domains:

- Communication with patients
- Information gathering
- Applied clinical knowledge
- Patient safety

The patient you are about to see has been referred to your outpatient department by her GP. Read the referral letter below and obtain relevant history from the patient and discuss what examination and test you feel are necessary with her. The examiner will inform you of the examination findings on request.

Dear colleague
Re. Mary Jones
I would be grateful if you could see this 26-year-old teacher who is complaining of intermenstrual bleeding. She is very anxious, and I would be grateful if you could see her.
Yours sincerely
Dr G Houston MRCGP

You have 10 minutes in which you should

- Take an appropriate history.
- Discuss appropriate examination and initial investigations.
- Discuss likely diagnoses and appropriate management options.

Simulated patient instructions

You are Mary Jones, a 26-year-old teacher in a stable relationship. You have been on the combined oral contraceptive pill (Microgynon) for 3 years and remember to take this as prescribed. You have no medical problems of note but smoke 15 cigarettes a day. You are nulliparous and have no immediate fertility plans but have had a first trimester surgical termination of pregnancy in the past.

Your menstrual cycles are regular and not heavy, but you have noticed light intermittent intermenstrual bleeding (spotting) over the past 6 months, which occurs at any time during the pill cycle. You have also noted some light bleeding after sexual intercourse on occasions recently. Although you have no pelvic pain or dyspareunia, you have noticed a heavy, clear, non-odorous vaginal discharge. You have never had a smear.

You are very worried about your symptoms, especially because your mother died 2 years ago from endometrial cancer.

If not discussed by the candidate, the following questions may be helpful:

- Why am I bleeding?
- What can I do to stop the bleeding?

Examiner instructions

Once the candidate begins to discuss which examinations they will perform, you can divulge the following examination findings:

Prominent cervical ectopy, friable but no cervical lesions. Otherwise normal lower genital tract and pelvis.

Marking

Communication with patient
- Adequate introduction, good body language with adequate eye contact.
- Able to describe the management plan and possible diagnosis clearly while avoiding medical jargon.
- Addresses concerns of patient in an empathetic manner.

Information gathering
- Takes a concise and relevant history.
- Requests appropriate investigations.
- Interprets the results of the examinations appropriately and develops a clear management plan with rationale.

Applied clinical knowledge
- The candidate should demonstrate knowledge of different causes for intermenstrual bleeding and arrange appropriate examination and investigations.
- An appropriate and well-thought-out management plan should be given.

Safety
- Cervical pathology should be considered as a cause of post-coital bleeding and examination, cervical smear, PID swabs and smoking cessation should be recommended.

Examiner notes

History

- Nature of IMB – Duration, pattern, timing, amount and frequency of bleeding, and also normal 'cycle' withdrawal bleeds
- COC and compliance
- Elicit PMB history and ascertain its nature – Amount, intermittent, not associated with dyspareunia
- Vaginal discharge
- Smear history and smoking
- Elicit TOP and family history

Examination and investigations

- Abdominal and pelvic examination
  - Inspection of the vulva/vagina (candida)
  - Inspection of cervix (ectopy, polyps, suspicious lesions, friability)
- Cervical smear
- Genital tract swabs
- Consider pelvic ultrasound

Diagnosis and management

- IMB – Breakthrough bleeding on COC but need to await swab results to exclude genital tract infection (*Chlamydia trachomatis*, candida, etc.).
- PCB – May be related to cervical ectopy but need to obtain smear result to exclude dyskaryosis and swabs to exclude genital tract infection.
- Vaginal discharge – Cervical ectopy, genital tract infection.
- Endometrial polyp.
- Reassure if tests are normal. Explain that cervical ectopy (exposed columnar cells) is physiological but can be more pronounced with the COC.
- Try changing COC to one with a different progestogen; consider Cerazette POP.
- Consider treatment of cervical ectopy (cauterisation or cryotherapy) only as second line as evidence of efficacy is limited.
- Treat genital tract infection appropriately with antibiotics, antifungals and arrange contact tracing via GU clinic if STI.
- Repeat smear±colposcopy if abnormal smear. Outpatient hysteroscopy and uterine polypectomy if polyp on scan.

Non-menstrual bleeding is common. Over a 6-month period, 7%–10% of women will experience IMB and 2%–4% PCB. Although the vast majority of women with unscheduled, non-menstrual bleeding do not have any significant underlying pathology, such symptoms tend to provoke a disproportionate amount of anxiety in patients and their doctors.

Routine referral is indicated for recurrent and persistent symptoms in association with a normal pelvic examination. Urgent referral should be considered where IMB/PCB symptoms are found in association with pelvic pain or dyspareunia or an abnormal pelvic examination (suspect appearance or lesions on vulva, vagina and cervix, friable cervix/contact bleeding, pelvic mass not thought to be fibroids) or abnormal cervical smear (squamous or glandular dyskaryosis, BNA, HPV, mild atypia on repeated testing).

There are many potential causes of IMB. However, in this case 'physiological bleeding' For example, mid-cycle–peri-ovulatory hormonal fluctuations (occurs in 1%–2% of normal cycles; luteal phase defect–inadequate progestogenic endometrial support) are not relevant because she is on the COC, and there is no cyclical pattern to IMB. Serious endometrial disease (cancer and hyperplasia) is unlikely in a woman under 40 years with regular cycles on the COC. Trauma and vulvo-vaginal pathology (urogenital atrophy, dermatoses, etc.) are unlikely causes of PCB in view of her age and absence of dyspareunia.

The main potential diagnoses are as follows:

1. Breakthrough bleeding in association with the COC, which is common initially even in women with good compliance and no drug interactions/GIT disorders.
2. Genital tract infection – Friable cervix may suggest cervicitis, past history of TOP and discharge (although malodorous and clearly suggests physiological).
3. Cervical dyskaryosis should be considered as a cause of PCB as she is over 25 years of age, has not had a cervical smear and is a smoker (*note*: up to 17% of women with PCB will have CIN).

Uterine polyps can cause endometrial dysregulation and lead to IMB/PCB, but this diagnosis is unlikely in women under 40 years with regular cycles. An ultrasound scan is relatively non-invasive and may be useful here to provide additional reassurance in view of her mother's history of uterine cancer. A hysteroscopy±endometrial biopsy is not indicated in view of the low prevalence of endometrial pathology, unless the scan reveals an abnormal endometrium.

Management will involve review of investigations and reassurance if all normal. As symptoms are not self-limiting (>6 months), it is reasonable to change the COC preparation to one with a different progestogen to see if it gives better endometrial support, absorption, etc. Although POPs are less effective than the COC and are associated with DUB, Cerazette POP prevents ovulation in 95% of women and so may provide better cycle control and the lack of exogenous oestrogen may reduce the size of the cervical ectopy.

Prominent cervical ectopies may be excised or ablated using a variety of outpatient methods and CIN treated by LLETZ. It should be noted, however, that although a modest association between presence of cervical ectopy and vaginal discharge has been shown, no such association has been found with PCB or IMB. Thus, such intervention, especially in young, nulliparous women, should be considered second line for refractory cases.

MODULE 12: EARLY PREGNANCY

Candidate instructions

This station is a structured VIVA and will assess your abilities to answer questions surrounding the management of ectopic pregnancy. You will be assessed using the following domains:

- Patient safety
- Communication with colleagues
- Information gathering
- Applied clinical knowledge

You are the O&G registrar on-call on the weekend. You are on labour ward when you are telephoned by the A+E Department. The A+E registrar tells you that there is a 21-year-old patient in their resuscitation area who has collapsed at home. She has a positive pregnancy test. Her mother has told the A+E team that she had been complaining of lower abdominal pain and then collapsed.

You will have 10 minutes to answer questions regarding your assessment and management of this patient. You will be assessed according to your ability in answering the questions and the amount of prompting that you require.

Marking

Patient safety

- Understands the risks of leaving the labour ward without calling for appropriate help.
- Demonstrates the need to take a quick history for a patient that is acutely unwell.
- Able to coordinate the emergency theatre team in order to facilitate safe surgical treatment for the patient.
- Understands the risks of choosing the correct surgical technique in a patient that is acutely unwell.
- Escalates to seniors appropriately.

Communication with colleagues

- Communicates clearly with the labour ward shift leader, CA+E team and the emergency theatre team to optimise the outcome for the patient.
- Provides structured answers to the questions asked.
- Justifies their choice of surgical technique.

Information gathering

- Collects clinical details from the labour ward before leaving to attend A+E.
- Gathers important information from the patient required to safely manage her ectopic pregnancy.

Applied clinical knowledge

- Demonstrates knowledge of initial resuscitation of the acutely unwell patient with a ruptured ectopic pregnancy.
- Demonstrates clinical knowledge regarding the safest surgical treatment for an unstable patient with a ruptured ectopic pregnancy.

Examiner notes

Ask the questions below to the candidate in the sequence provided.

1. What further questions would you ask of the A+E registrar on the telephone?
   - Some further information regarding the cardiovascular state of the patient and other observations to gauge the urgency for your assessment and management.
   - Have they commenced initial resuscitation?
   - Have they cross-matched any blood products?
   - Have they notified the emergency theatre team and department already?
2. Before leaving the labour ward, what would you do?
   - Discuss the situation with your team, including the labour ward shift leader and your junior colleague/s.
   - Go through the labour ward board with the labour ward staff to ensure the safety of the patients that are present on the labour ward.
   - Inform the consultant on-call of the situation on delivery suite and the events in A+E. Ask for them to be on-site if they are not already.
   - Leave contact information for the labour ward shift leader to contact you if you are required back in an emergency.
3. You arrive in the A+E department. How would you assess the patient?
   - The candidate should make a brief assessment of the patient to understand the urgency of intervention using an ABC approach and also request observations including RR, O2 Saturations, BP, Pulse rate, capillary refill time, AVPU assessment.
   - If the candidate mentions that they would like to know the observations, provide the following information:
     - RR 23 bpm
     - O_2 saturations 98% on 7LO2
     - BP 96/63
     - P 134
     - CRT 4 seconds
     - Alert on AVPU scale
   - The candidate should mention that their concern is of a ruptured ectopic pregnancy in view of the clinical history that was relayed from the A+E registrar.
   - If possible, a quick and concise history should be obtained. This should include PC, HPC, LMP, PMH, PSH, DH, allergies, time last ate and drank.
   - An assessment of the patient's abdomen should be made. If this is mentioned, tell the candidate that the abdomen is distended and peritonitic.

4. Tell the candidate, 'The patient tells you that her LMP was 6 weeks ago, she has severe abdominal pain and that she is otherwise fit and well. She takes no regular medications and has no allergies'.

   In view of your assessment, what do you think is the most likely diagnosis?
   - Ruptured ectopic pregnancy with a substantial intra-abdominal bleed.

5. How would you now manage the patient?
   - Escalate the findings to the consultant on-call.
   - Make provisions for emergency surgical management of ruptured ectopic pregnancy.
   - Take blood tests for FBC, U+E. Cross match 2–4 units of blood.
   - Inform the on-call anaesthetist and theatre team.
   - Do not perform imaging as the patient is acutely unwell.
   - Consent the patient for surgical treatment of ruptured ectopic pregnancy. Inform the patient that this could be via laparoscopy or laparotomy. The candidate should justify whichever route. Ideally, this patient would undergo a laparotomy in view of her unstable cardiovascular status.
   - Transfer the patient immediately to the emergency theatre.

6. You successfully manage her ruptured ectopic pregnancy in the emergency theatre with the help of your consultant by performing an open salpingectomy. She had 1.5 L of blood in her abdomen and was transfused 2 units of blood. She will return to the gynaecology ward after her recovery from anaesthetic. What should you do now?
   - Complete your operation notes.
   - Inform the shift leader on labour ward of your imminent return and ensure the safety of the patients on labour ward.
   - Take the next available opportunity to debrief the patient explaining your intraoperative findings and management – likely salpingectomy.
   - Ensure that she is prescribed post-operative medications including thromboprophylaxis and analgesia.
   - Counsel her with regard to the implications of her ruptured ectopic pregnancy. This should include the need for early ultrasound scans in subsequent pregnancies and impact on future fertility.

Revision notes

Occasionally, in the MRCOG Part 3 exam you will be expected to demonstrate that you are able to manage multiple clinical scenarios at once. This is truly reflective of clinical practice, and the RCOG would be examining your ability to multitask whilst ensuring that the patients under your care are kept safe. Patient safety is key in this scenario, it is tempting to go and manage the collapsed patient in the A+E department. However, it is also imperative that you also ensure the ongoing safety of the patients that you are caring for on the labour ward. What is being assessed are the soft skills required to manage a team effectively and your skills at communicating and escalating appropriately with the multidisciplinary team members.

MODULE 13: ONCOLOGY

Candidate instructions

This station is with a simulated patient and will assess the following domains:

- Information gathering
- Communication with patients
- Applied clinical knowledge
- Patient safety

You have been asked to see Judith Davies, a 62-year-old who has been referred by her GP. She presented with abdominal bloating so he arranged a pelvic and abdominal ultrasound and serum CA125.The serum CA125 level was 45. The pelvic and abdominal ultrasound showed an 11cm multilocular cyst on the left ovary with solid areas. The right ovary and uterus was normal. There was no free fluid in the pouch of Douglas. The liver was not normal; there was no other abnormality of note.

You have 10 minutes to do the following:

1. Take a relevant history.
2. Explain the investigation findings.
3. Formulate and explain a management plan to the patient.
4. Answer any questions the patient has.

Simulated patient instructions

You are Judith Davies, a 62-year-old business manager. You live with your husband Mario an accountant and your 21-year-old daughter who is a full-time student.

You presented to the GP because you were feeling tired and had abdominal bloating for the last 3 months. You have no other bowel or urinary symptoms. You have not noticed any weight change. Your GP arranged a blood test and a scan; you do not know the results of these investigations.

You went through the menopause when you were 56 years old. The only pregnancy you have had was your daughter who was conceived via IVF and delivered at term with a vaginal delivery. You have never had any abnormal smear tests.

You have an active lifestyle and do not drink or smoke. You have never had any surgery or serious medical problems. You are not taking any medication and have no allergies. Your mother died of breast cancer when she was 40 years old.

You have heard there is an association between breast cancer and ovarian cancer and are very worried about the risk to your daughter.

If not discussed by the candidate, the following questions may be useful:

- Do I have cancer/what are the chances of cancer?
- What happens next?
- Is my daughter at risk of cancer?

Marking

Information gathering

- The candidate should take a relevant history.
- The investigations should be interpreted correctly.

Communication with patients

- Deals with the patient sensitively and offers to meet again with their partner or friend.
- Uses appropriate warning shot(s) before breaking bad news and gives time after to allow the information to sink in.
- Give the patient information in manageable amounts and deals sensitively with and questions.
- The candidate describes the management plan clearly.

Applied clinical knowledge

- The candidate should be able to use the data to formulate an appropriate management plan.
- They should appreciate and convey to the patient that further imaging (CT) is needed before definitive management plan can be made during a gynaecology oncology MDT.
- They should give a brief description of the gynaecology oncology MDT.

Patient safety

- The candidate should recognise the risk of ovarian cancer and have an appropriate management plan.
- There should be an understanding of the correct referral pathways and treatment targets.

Examiner notes

A directed history should explore ovarian cancer-related symptoms such as bowel problems, bloating, appetite and weight loss. They should identify the patient risk factors for surgery by determining if there are any medical problems, previous surgery and smoking status. The candidate should build a picture of the patients social support network (e.g. who does she live with).The history should identify her mother died of breast cancer and this could mean there is *BRCA* gene in the family. It is important not to get drawn into an in-depth conversation about hereditary gynaecological cancers at this point, but it is important to respond to patient concerns. It is thought that around 20% of epithelial ovarian cancers are hereditary. At this point, it is not certain that there is a cancer and if it contains a *BRCA* gene mutation. A lot more extra information will be gathered once the cyst is removed. Referral can then be made to a regional genetic centre for further information and counselling.

During the 2-minute preparation time, the candidate should work out the risk of malignancy to determine further management. According to the RCOG greentop guideline for the management of ovarian cysts in postmenopausal women, this should be done with the Risk of Malignancy Index (RMI).The RMI I combines the three features: the serum CA125 level, the menopausal status (M) and the ultrasound score (U).The menopausal status is scored as 1 for premenopausal women and 3 for postmenopausal women. The ultrasound score gets one point for each of the following: metastases, solid areas, multilocular cysts, ascites and lesions. The ultrasound score is 0 for 0 points; 1 for 1 points and 3 for 2–5 points. In this case, the RMI I score is as follows:

$$U \times M \times CA125 = RMI \cdot I$$

$$3 \text{ (for multilocular cyst with solid areas)} \times 3 \text{ (postmenopausal)} \times 45 = 405$$

As the RMI I is ≥200, there is increased risk of malignancy. This means further imaging in the form of a CT abdomen and pelvis, and a referral to gynaecological oncology MDT should be arranged. If the MDT determines there is a high likelihood of malignancy, then she will need a full staging laparotomy; if they decide there is low likelihood of malignancy, then she will need a TAH + BSO + omentectomy + peritoneal cytology.

With the RMI score being greater than 250, the risk of cancer is around 75%. It is important to prepare and give correct information. In real practice, you would study the notes, discuss the case with relevant colleagues and find out as much as you can about the condition (prognosis, management and support). It is important to resist the temptation to guess at information you do not know.

Although we do not have a diagnosis, the results of the investigation will come as bad news to most patients. It is important to play it straight and tell the patient there is risk of cancer after an appropriate warning shot. For example, 'I'm afraid the investigations do not show good news (warning shot).The scan and blood test show there is a risk of ovarian cancer'. It is important to give the patient time to digest the information and respond to their queries. It might mean repeating the information. At this stage, the candidate should not get drawn into giving detailed prognostic information but can give appropriate hope.

Further reading: RCOG Scientific Impact Paper No 48 Management of Women with Genetic Predisposition of Gynaecological Cancers and RCOG green-top guideline for the management of ovarian cysts in postmenopausal women.

MODULE 14: UROGYNAECOLOGY AND THE PELVIC FLOOR

Candidate instructions

This station is a role-play station and will assess your ability to take a clinical history from the patient and then discuss the management options. You are the gynaecology registrar in a urogynaecology out-patients clinic. You are to see Mrs. Eva Grey, a 56-year-old woman who has been having some incontinence of urine.

She has undergone some urodynamic studies as she was having some mixed urinary incontinence symptoms. The urodynamics read out is shown in Figure 11.3.

You are to discuss with Mrs. Grey what has been shown formulate a management plan for her given her clinical details.

You will be assessed using the following domains:

- Patient safety
- Communication with patients and their relatives
- Information gathering
- Applied clinical knowledge

You will have 10 minutes to discuss the findings of her urodynamics study, take a history and to discuss her ongoing management plan.

Simulated patient instructions

You are Eva Grey, a 56-year-old managing director of a printing company. You have been leaking urine for the past 8 months and your symptoms are getting worse. Occasionally, you leak on sneezing but this has happened ever since the birth of your third child. Things have come to a head recently as you are finding that you have to run to the toilet during meetings and there have been a couple of incidents when you did not make it on time. These symptoms are getting in the way of your work and you wish to have them treated. It is getting embarrassing having to make excuses to your work colleagues before running out of the meeting room. You have no symptoms of prolapse.

You have had three children before, all by C/S. Apart from the three caesarean sections, you have not had any other surgery. You went through the menopause at

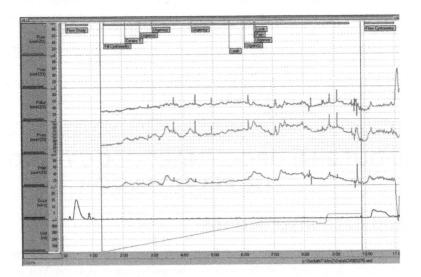

Figure 11.3 Urodynamics of Eva Grey.

age 48 and have had no post-menopausal bleeding. Your smears are up to date and you have had one loop excision of your cervix when you are around 35 years old.

You are otherwise fit and well and do not take any regular medications. You have no allergies and do not smoke or drink alcohol. You do enjoy your coffee, drinking five cups per day, mainly in the morning. You live with your husband Brian and your three children. You remain sexually active but recently you have not had a great libido due to the fact that you keep on leaking urine and running to the toilet.

If not covered by the candidate, questions that you could ask include:

- What is detrusor overactivity?
- Why have I started to have the symptoms now?
- What treatments are available for me?
- How long does it usually take for the symptoms to improve after starting the tablets?
- What are the side effects if I choose to take the tablet medications?
- Is there anything else that I can do to help my symptoms?

Marking

Patient safety
- Interprets data from the urodynamics study correctly.
- Correctly identifies that the report belongs to Mrs Grey.
- Takes a full history so that use of anti-muscarinics treatment is safe.
- Checks allergy history.

Communication with patients and their relatives
- Explains the findings of the urodynamic study without jargon.
- Explains the concept of detrusor overactivity well – may use a diagram as an aid.
- Listens attentively to the patient as they explain the symptoms that they have been experiencing.
- Explains the management options so that they are simple to understand.
- Ends the consultation appropriately.

Information gathering
- Interprets the urodynamic study correctly.
- Gathers a concise urogynaecology history from the patient.
- Gathers information from the patient that may be important for urinary incontinence and information that may preclude the use of antimuscarinic therapy.

Applied clinical knowledge
- Makes the correct diagnosis of detrusor overactivity.
- Able to interpret the urodynamic study accurately.
- Understands the risk factors for stress and urge urinary incontinence.
- Demonstrates understanding of the NICE incontinence guideline.

Examiner notes

- The candidate identify that the urodynamic study belongs to Mrs Grey.
- The candidate should demonstrate to Mrs Grey what the urodynamic shows – detrusor activity with urinary incontinence.
- The candidate should find out what symptoms Mrs Grey has been experiencing.
- The candidate should take a quick concise history from the patient. This should include the following:
  - PC
  - HPC with caffeine intake, fluid intake, other urinary symptoms, bowel symptoms, sexual symptoms, smear history, menopausal history
  - PMH
  - PSH
  - POH
  - DH/allergies
  - SH
  - FH
- The candidates should explain that the first course of action now that detrusor overactivity has been confirmed is to ensure that lifestyle measures are implemented – weight loss if applicable, reduce caffeine and fluid intake.
- Pelvic floor exercises should be arranged for Mrs Grey if not already organised as she has mixed symptoms.
- Bladder training exercises should be organised for 6 weeks.
- The candidate should start some antimuscarinic therapy. It is acceptable if the candidate does not know the exact dose or timing of administration but they should show that they would check with a senior or consult the BNF.
- The following antimuscarinic agents can be offered:
  - Oxybutynin
  - Tolterodine
  - Darifenacin
- The candidate could offer a patient information leaflet regarding antimuscarinic therapy.
- The side effects of dry mouth and constipation.
- Follow-up should be at around 4 weeks after commencement of treatment as this is when any benefit from the drug treatment will be experienced.

INDEX